T0358755

Curbside Consultation
in GERD

49 Clinical Questions

CURBSIDE CONSULTATION IN GASTROENTEROLOGY
SERIES

SERIES EDITOR, FRANCIS A. FARRAYE, MD, MSc, FACP, FACG

Curbside Consultation
in GERD
49 Clinical Questions

Philip O. Katz, MD. FACG

Chairman, Division of Gastroenterology
Albert Einstein Medical Center
Clinical Professor of Medicine
Jefferson Medical College
Philadelphia, PA

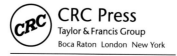

CRC Press
Taylor & Francis Group
Boca Raton London New York

CRC Press is an imprint of the
Taylor & Francis Group, an **informa** business

First published 2008 by SLACK Incorporated

Published 2024 by CRC Press
2385 NW Executive Center Drive, Suite 320, Boca Raton FL 33431

and by CRC Press
4 Park Square, Milton Park, Abingdon, Oxon, OX14 4RN

CRC Press is an imprint of Taylor & Francis Group, LLC

© 2008 Taylor & Francis Group, LLC

Library of Congress Cataloging-in-Publication Data

Katz, Philip O., 1953-
    Curbside consultation in GERD : 49 clinical questions / Philip Katz.
      p. ; cm.
    Includes bibliographical references.
    ISBN-13: 9781556428180 (alk. paper)
    1. Gastroesophageal reflux--Miscellanea. I. Title.
    [DNLM: 1. Gastroesophageal Reflux. WI 250 K19c 2008]

RC815.7.K38 2008
616.3'24--dc22
                                2008000126

ISBN: 9781556428180 (pbk)
ISBN: 9781003523529 (ebk)

DOI: 10.1201/9781003523529

Dedication

This book is dedicated to my mother, Marilyn Katz. Her unwavering support and strength have helped me immeasurably throughout my life and career. Without her, none of this would be possible.

Contents

Contents

Contents

Acknowledgments

Thanks to my long time administrative assistant, Debbie Bruestle. I could not and would not have done this without her skill.

Special thanks to Leilani for supporting this and all of my professional ventures.

About the Author

Philip O. Katz, MD is Chairman of the Division of Gastroenterology at Albert Einstein Medical Center and Clinical Professor of Medicine at Jefferson Medical College in Philadelphia, PA. He is also Associate Program Director of the Department of Medicine at Albert Einstein Medical Center.

Dr. Katz received his medical degree from the Bowman Gray School of Medicine at Wake Forest University in Winston-Salem, NC. He served his residency and chief residency in internal medicine, followed by a fellowship in gastroenterology at the Bowman Gray School of Medicine. He completed a faculty development fellowship at Johns Hopkins University in Baltimore, MD. He is board certified in internal medicine and gastroenterology.

Dr. Katz is currently Vice President of the American College of Gastroenterology and is a member of the American Gastroenterological Association and the American Society for Gastrointestinal Endoscopy.

A recognized national authority on esophageal disease, Dr. Katz's research interests include all aspects of gastroesophageal reflux disease, including nocturnal recovery of gastric acid secretion during proton pump inhibitor therapy and esophageal pain perception. Dr. Katz is a practicing clinician with active teaching and editorial positions. In addition to lecturing on many gastroenterology-related topics, Dr. Katz is Associate Editor for *Reviews in Gastrointestinal Disorders* (Med Reviews) and an editorial reviewer for *Annals of Internal Medicine, American Journal of Gastroenterology, Gastroenterology,* and *Digestive Diseases and Sciences.* He has contributed to the publication of over 120 peer-reviewed papers as well as numerous abstracts, books, book chapters, and monographs.

MR. SMITH IS A 52-YEAR-OLD MAN WHO HAS NEVER BEEN ON PPI THERAPY. AFTER AN ED VISIT FOR CHEST PAIN, HE IS FOUND TO HAVE GRADE D EROSIVE ESOPHAGITIS. I HAVE STARTED OMEPRAZOLE 40 MG DAILY, AND HIS SYMPTOMS HAVE RESOLVED. DOES HE NEED A FOLLOW-UP ENDOSCOPY?

This 52-year-old man with presumed gastroesophageal reflux disease, erosive esophagitis grade D, is referred for a question related to the need for follow-up endoscopy. In order to answer this question in the most efficient manner, there are several bits of information that would be helpful. I have been given little background on the patient. Specifically whether or not he is presenting with chest pain for the first time; whether he has heartburn, regurgitation, or any other symptom of gastroesophageal reflux disease; and/or whether he has had any other treatment for GERD. It would be unusual for a 52-year-old man to present with chest pain as his sole symptom for GERD having no other symptoms or other past intervention. Nevertheless, for the purpose of answering this question, I will assume that he has had cardiac disease ruled out, which is mandatory for a gastroenterologist managing a patient with chest pain, a thorough history taken, and as such underwent endoscopy for evaluation of the chest pain.

Figure 1-1. Grade D erosive esophagitis. This photo is meant to illustrate the Los Angeles classification of erosive esophagitis. Using this system, it is highly unlikely that grades A and B erosions would obscure any but the shortest segments of columnar lining, but grades C and D might. It is in the latter that repeat endoscopy might be considered.

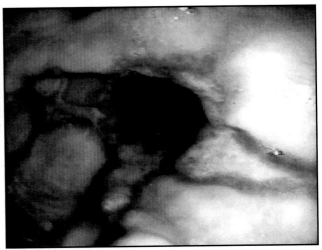

The use of endoscopy as an evaluative tool in patients with unexplained chest pain is, to some degree, debated. Although it appears to be the usual first diagnostic test in the community, the "yield" of this intervention is not nearly as high as it would be had this patient presented with frequent heartburn. Chest pain literature for the most part suggests that erosive esophagitis is seen in a minority, about 10% to 15%, which is in keeping with my clinical experience. A well-done study from the Veterans Administration in Tucson, Arizona, found the frequency of erosive esophagitis to be higher (35%) than other studies in the literature, and a recent report (personal communication) of a large endoscopic database found that endoscopic abnormalities are seen in 25% to 35% of patients endoscoped when noncardiac chest pain is listed as the reason for endoscopy. In addition, the finding of grade D erosive esophagitis (the most severe on the A, B, C, D grading system; Figure 1-1) is in my experience quite unusual in patients with non-cardiac chest pain. A therapeutic trial of high dose proton pump inhibitor is the most efficient and cost-effective approach to this patient.

Although it is likely that the erosive esophagitis is due to gastroesophageal reflux disease, it would be imperative to be certain that the patient had no history of pill ingestion that might contribute to esophagitis nor any history in which one might develop infectious esophagitis that might confuse the picture. Assuming this is grade D erosive esophagitis secondary to reflux, the determination of follow-up endoscopy in my practice is based on a single question. Should this patient be screened for Barrett's esophagus and is his initial endoscopy sufficient to rule that out? As I will discuss in other questions, the risks for Barrett's esophagus are the following: Caucasian, male, long history of reflux symptoms (greater than 5 to 10 years), and early onset of reflux symptoms (prior to age 35). I know only that he is 52 years old. Given the absence of this history, let's presume that he is in a high-risk category and therefore is a candidate for screening. It is clear from my own observations that a columnar lined esophagus can be obscured by severe erosive esophagitis and that inflammation on biopsy may obscure accurate interpretation of the histologic findings. There are no well-designed studies, however, that support this observation so an argument for follow-up endoscopy could not be made based purely on the available evidence or data. However, it would be my preference to electively re-endoscope the patient to be certain that he did not have Barrett's even in the absence of any symptoms. It would not be necessary to endoscope this patient purely to document healing as there is little evidence, if any, that his disease would progress to further complications should he not heal, in the absence of Barrett's metaplasia.

Clinicians can be comfortable that in the absence of Barrett's, there is little reason to believe that erosive esophagitis is an independent risk for complications or will progress to Barrett's. As such, healing itself does not need to be documented to optimally manage GERD symptoms.

Bibliography

Fass R, Fennerty MB, Ofman JJ, et al. The clinical and economic value of a short course of omeprazole in patients with noncardiac chest pain. *Gastroenterology.* 1998;115(1):42-49.

Pandak WM, Arezo S, Everett S, et al. Short course of omeprazole: a better first diagnostic approach to noncardiac chest pain than endoscopy, manometry, or 24-hour esophageal pH monitoring. *J Clin Gastroenterol.* 2002;35(4):307-314.

QUESTION

WHAT ARE THE INDICATIONS FOR ENDOSCOPY IN PATIENTS WITH CLASSIC GASTROESOPHAGEAL REFLUX DISEASE?

There are no absolute indications for endoscopy in patients with classic gastroesophageal reflux disease. In order to answer this question, one again must assume that classic gastroesophageal reflux disease means that the patient has 1 or 2 primary symptoms: heartburn and/or regurgitation. In this setting, the approach to consideration of upper gastrointestinal (GI) endoscopy is based on guidelines, and patient preference. If the disease is uncomplicated—heartburn and/or regurgitation as the only symptom, easily resolved with antisecretory therapy—then endoscopy is purely elective and I would discuss the risks and benefits based on the risk profile for Barrett's esophagus (see below). I tend to be aggressive in screening patients for Barrett's because I believe that the approach to the patient is subtly different with and without Barrett's esophagus. However, one could argue based on the evidence in the literature that there is no indication to screen or endoscope a patient who is asymptomatic on antisecretory therapy. So, I would have a discussion with the patient and be most inclined to endoscope this patient if he were Caucasian, male, over the age of 50, and had reflux symptoms for more than 5 to 10 years. If this was not a description of our patient, I would offer a screening examination but would be less inclined to "push it" in any way. I do my Barrett's screening endoscopy after at least 8 weeks of antisecretory therapy in attempt to make certain the mucosa is healed prior to endoscopy. If the patient had classic reflux symptoms and had not responded to antisecretory therapy, I would perform endoscopy for diagnostic purposes to determine if there was another problem related to the symptoms. If the patient had any of the so-called alarm symptoms, dysphagia, odynophagia (painful swallowing), weight loss, anemia, or other signs of a systemic process, then I would consider an endoscopy prior to instituting a therapeutic trial. I do not consider chest pain, cough, or

Figure 2-1. Endoscopic findings in 97 patients presenting with reflux symptoms 3 times a week for greater than 5 years indicate that many patients with heartburn may have a normal endoscopy. As such, it is often recommended that a therapeutic trial of antisecretory therapy precede endoscopy in the absence of alarm symptoms. (Reprinted from Winters C, Spurling TJ, Chobanina SJ, et al. Barrett's esophagus: a prevalent, occult complication of gastroesophageal reflux disease. *Gastroenterology.* 1987;92:118-124, with permission from Elsevier.)

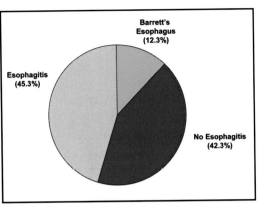

Table 2-1

Role of Endoscopy in GERD

- Make a diagnosis
- Rule out complications
- Grade disease severity
- Influence management?
  * Up to 50% of people with heartburn do not have visible findings
  * Severity of heartburn does not predict presence of esophagitis
  * Lack of esophagitis does not predict easier-to-treat subset of patients

Katz PO. Treatment of gastroesophageal reflux disease: use of algorithms to aid in management. *Am J Gastroenterol.* 1999;94:S3-S10.
DeVault KR, Castell DO. American College of Gastroenterology. Updated guidelines for the diagnosis and treatment of gastroesophageal reflux disease. *Am J Gastroenterol.* 2005;100(1):190-200.

asthma a warning (alarm) sign. It is important to remember that endoscopy is limited in sensitivity in the diagnosis of GERD so a normal exam does rule out the disease and an abnormal exam does not guarantee that GERD is the cause for symptoms (Figure 2-1). The ACG Guidelines for endoscopy are outlined Tables 2-1 and 2-2.

Bibliography

DeVault KR, Castell DO. American College of Gastroenterology. Updated guidelines for the diagnosis and treatment of gastroesophageal reflux disease. *Am J Gastroenterol.* 2005;100(1):190-200.

Sampliner RE. Practice Parameters Committee of the American College of Gastroenterology. Updated guidelines for the diagnosis, surveillance, and therapy of Barrett's esophagus. *Am J Gastroenterol.* 2002;97(8):1888-1895.

Winters C, Spurling TJ, Chobanina SJ, et al. Barrett's esophagus: a prevalent, occult complication of gastroesophageal reflux disease. *Gastroenterology.* 1987;92:118-124.

<u>Table 2-2</u>

General Guidelines for Appropriate use of Endoscopy in GERD

- For patients with uncomplicated GERD
  - * Initial trial of empiric therapy
  - * Endoscopy if empiric therapy unsuccessful or if symptoms recur after initial response
- Endoscopy
  - * Promptly indicated with warning symptoms of cancer or infection
    - o Dysphagia, odynophagia, weight loss, bleeding, blood in stool, anemia, persistent vomiting
  - * Recommended with symptoms for >5 years to rule out Barrett's esophagus
    - Render asymptomatic for 8 weeks before testing

DeVault KR, Castell DO. American College of Gastroenterology. Updated guidelines for the diagnosis and treatment of gastroesophageal reflux disease. *Am J Gastroenterol.* 2005;100(1):190-200. Sampliner RE. Practice Parameters Committee of the American College of Gastroenterology. Updated guidelines for the diagnosis, surveillance, and therapy of Barrett's esophagus. *Am J Gastroenterol.* 2002;97(8):1888-1895.

Ms. Jones Is a 45-Year-Old School Teacher Who Has Reflux Controlled on BID Omeprazole. She Does Not Like to Take Medications and Would Like to Consider Fundoplication. Is This Reasonable Given Her Good Response To PPI Therapy?

This 45-year-old patient asks about the possibility of a fundoplication (antireflux surgery). She does not wish to take antisecretory therapy long term; one of several reasons patients have surgery (Figure 3-1). We are told she has had a good response to proton pump inhibitor (PPI) therapy and that she has reflux. This is a reasonable time to consider antireflux surgery. In my practice, there are no absolute indications for surgery. I often stress to students, residents, and other colleagues that the best reason to perform antireflux surgery is in the patient who does not want to take medicine long term, has proven gastroesophageal reflux disease (GERD) and has responded to a trial of medical therapy (preferably asymptomatic). As such, we need to be absolutely certain that this patient has GERD. I would not be comfortable with the diagnosis if the only evaluation was a history, physical, and therapeutic trial. If I see a patient who has been treated empirically and surgery is being considered, the patient would have endoscopy, pH monitoring, and a preop esophageal function evaluation (esophageal manometry) to determine if indeed she had

Reason*	Patients (%)
Medications did not work	46
Physician recommended it	45
Thought it would cure the disease	27
Did not wish to take medications for long term	15
High cost of medications	4
To prevent cancer	3

N = 80
*Some patients reported more than one reason

Figure 3-1. Why patients choose surgery? Many patients had more than 1 reason, many of which I do not consider good reasons to operate. Patients should be clear that no therapy, including surgery, will reliably prevent cancer. (Reprinted from Vakil N, Shaw M, Kirby R. Clinical effectiveness of laparoscopic fundoplication in a U.S. community. *Am J Med.* 2003;114:1-5, with permission from Excerpta Medica.)

GERD and that there were no issues related to performing the fundoplication.

Many still believe that patients should have surgery when they are nonresponders to PPI. It is very clear from the literature and my personal experience that the best responders to antireflux surgery are those that have gastroesophageal reflux disease, a good to excellent response to antisecretory therapy, an abnormal pH study (Table 3-1), and do not have coexistent functional gastrointestinal disease. The former can be based on the literature as well as personal observations. The latter is a personal observation from my practice. Specifically, patients with irritable bowel syndrome and/or coexistent functional dyspepsia more often have residual symptoms after antireflux surgery and in my personal experience are not as happy. Nevertheless, if they understand the risks and benefits of the procedure, they would still be candidates.

Though overall, patients with atypical symptoms of GERD have a poorer response to surgery, the good response to PPI is key. If they respond to a PPI trial, they should do well at surgery. Patients who have not responded to a PPI should be evaluated thoroughly to determine the reasons. As PPI resistance is extremely rare, few will truly "fail a PPI" because of failure to control intragastric pH (acid). Usually "failure" is because symptoms are due to something other than acid. Nevertheless, to be certain that pH control on PPI is adequate, I always perform intragastric pH studies (combined with an assessment of esophageal reflux) in patients considering surgery who are PPI nonresponders. If they still have acid reflux and do not wish to consider further medical treatment I will refer to surgical evaluation. If non-acid reflux is believed to be the "cause" for symptoms, I will discuss surgery with the patient knowing that outcomes studies are limited in these patients.

Table 3-1

Predictors of Surgical Success

- GERD is proven
- Patient has responded to PPI
- Typical symptoms
- Experienced surgeon

Bibiography

Jackson PG, Gleiber MA, Askari R, Evans SR. Predictors of outcome in 100 consecutive laparoscopic antireflux procedures. *Am J Surg.* 2001;181:231-235.

Vakil N, Shaw M, Kirby R. Clinical effectiveness of laparoscopic fundoplication in a U.S. community. *Am J Med.* 2003;114:1-5.

HOW IMPORTANT IS SURGEON SELECTION IN ANTIREFLUX SURGERY? IS THE LAPAROSCOPIC APPROACH NOW STANDARD OF CARE FOR A NISSEN FUNDOPLICATION?

The decision to undergo antireflux surgery is complex. Medical therapy in and of itself if successful is an excellent long-term option with documented long-term success, usually at a stable dose of medication, with little to no long-term risk. Although there have been recent concerns about the possibility of enteric infections, pneumonia, and most recently hip fractures in patients taking long-term proton pump inhibitors, in general I do not believe any of these are reasons to consider surgery. Because there are potential complications of an elective operation, I believe that surgical selection is the key to optimal outcomes for this procedure and supported by consensus guidelines (Textboxes 4-1 and 4-2). In my years of practice, the patients seem happier when they have been operated on by an experienced esophageal surgeon, or a general surgeon who makes foregut surgery a regular part of their practice, seem to have less complicated postoperative course, and a better symptomatic outcome. Although clearly a "bias," those seen in my practice for complications of antireflux surgery appear to be from surgeons who do not do the operation frequently. There are no "numbers" that speaks to which surgeon is qualified, so the gastroenterologist needs to ask about experience and training and about surgical results and consider watching a surgeon operate if they have concerns about qualifications. Experienced antireflux surgeons are comfortable with the challenges often encountered in this operation, especially in those with complex disease. Conversion to open surgery is lower with an experienced surgeon, as is operative time and length of hospital stay (Figures 4-1 and 4-2).

Textbox 4-1

Surgical Therapy for GERD

- Critical Factors
  - * Careful preoperative assessment of patient
  - * Expertise of surgeon (learning curve)
- Positive response to medical therapy is the best predictor of successful surgical outcome

DeVault KR, Castell DO. Updated guidelines for the diagnosis and treatment of gastroesophageal reflux disease. *Am J Gastroenterol.* 2005;100(1):190-200.
So JBY, Zeitels SM, Rattner DW. Outcomes of atypical symptoms attributed to gastroesophageal reflux treated by laparoscopic fundoplication. *Surgery.* 1998;124:28-32.

Textbox 4-2

Antireflux Surgery Guidelines

- Antireflux surgery, performed by an experienced surgeon, is a maintenance option for the patient with well-documented GERD.
- The choice between medical and surgical therapy should depend upon informed patient preference.

Dent J, Brun J, Fendrick AM, et al. An evidence-based appraisal of reflux disease management --- the Genval Workshop Report. *Gut.* 1999;44(suppl 2):S1-S16.
DeVault KR, Castell DO. Updated guidelines for the diagnosis and treatment of gastroesophageal reflux disease. *Am J Gastroenterol.* 2005;100(1):190-200.

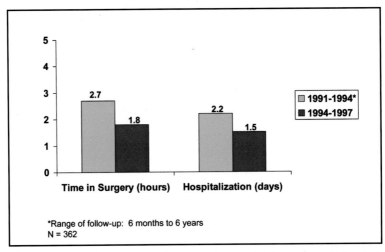

Figure 4-1. Results of increasing experience with laparoscopic fundoplication on length of operation and length of hospital stay. (Reprinted from Frantzides CT, Richards C. A study of 362 consecutive laparoscopic Nissen fundoplications. *Surgery.* 1998;124:651-654, with permission from Elsevier.)

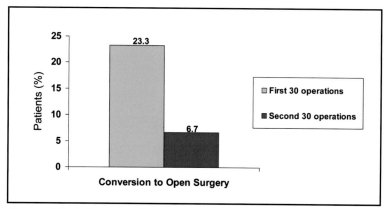

Figure 4-2. Influence of surgeon experience in laparoscopic fundoplication. Even though an early study in the laparoscopic era, this clearly indicates a "learning" curve for fundoplication. (Reprinted from Deschamps C, Allen MS, Trastek VF, et al. Early experience and learning curve associated with laparoscopic Nissen fundoplication. *J Thorac Cardiovasc Surg.* 1998;15:281-284, with permission from Elsevier.)

Laparoscopic antireflux surgery has been performed world wide since the early 1990s, has equivalent efficacy to open fundoplication, and results in substantially lower morbidity (shorter postoperative course, quicker return to normal activity, less postoperative discomfort). There are some data in the literature that indicate that the laparoscopic approach may increase the frequency of postoperative dysphagia. This is not a complication that I have seen in my experience. Therefore, I believe that when technically feasible, the laparoscopic approach should be used for all patients electing a Nissen fundoplication. Open surgery should be performed only when the laparoscopic approach is not feasible or a complex operation is required. This may include a patient with a very short esophagus or a patient who has had multiple fundoplications and requires revision. These decisions are always left to the surgeon performing the procedure.

Bibliography

DeVault KR, Castell DO. American College of Gastroenterology. Updated guidelines for the diagnosis and treatment of gastroesophageal reflux disease. *Am J Gastroenterol.* 2005;100(1):190-200.

Deschamps C, Allen MS, Trastek VF, et al. Early experience and learning curve associated with laparoscopic Nissen fundoplication. *J Thorac Cardiovasc Surg.* 1998;15:281-284.

Frantzides CT, Richards C. A study of 362 consecutive laparoscopic Nissen fundoplications. *Surgery.* 1998;124: 651-654.

A 55-Year-Old Man Is Referred for Evaluation for Antireflux Surgery. What Is the Appropriate Preoperative Evaluation of This Patient? Is Esophageal Function Testing (Manometry) Needed?

When considering antireflux surgery in a patient with GERD, the key preoperative questions are these:

1. Has gastroesophageal reflux disease been accurately and effectively documented?

2. Has a proton pump inhibitor trial been done? If so, what were the results? In effect, the success of a proton pump inhibitor therapeutic trial remains one of the best preoperative evaluation tools in this gentleman. It is noted elsewhere in the book that a successful proton pump inhibitor trial is the key to predicting success for antireflux surgery.

3. Has a preoperative evaluation been performed? Has endoscopy been performed? Although not mandatory, a preoperative endoscopic examination affords the opportunity to screen for Barrett's esophagus. Although the presence of Barrett's should not directly effect decisions for surgery, postoperative surveillance will be important and therefore appropriate Barrett's length and assessment for dysplasia are pertinent prior to surgery. In addition, many feel (and I agree) that there is a decrease in response, that there is a lower success rate for antireflux surgery in

the presence of Barrett's. Further, surgery has its best success in patients without erosions so if erosive esophagitis remains, I would be more aggressive with my antireflux medical therapy prior to operation. It is my preference to perform pre-op, prolonged pH monitoring as this will establish without question, the diagnosis of GERD and allow for understanding of the potential pathophysiology of symptom recurrence after surgery should that occur.

Though the literature debates the value of preoperative esophageal function testing (esophageal manometry) in predicting surgical success (Table 5-1) and/or tailoring

Table 5-1
Clinical Indications for Esophageal Manometry

- Evaluation of patients with dysphagia
  - * Primary motility disorders
    - o Achalasia
    - o Spastic disorders
  - * Secondary motility disorders
    - o Scleroderma
- Evaluation of patients with GERD
  - * Evaluate peristalsis and LES
    - o GERD severity
    - o Prior to fundoplication
  - * Assist in placement of pH probe
- Evaluation of patients with noncardiac chest pain

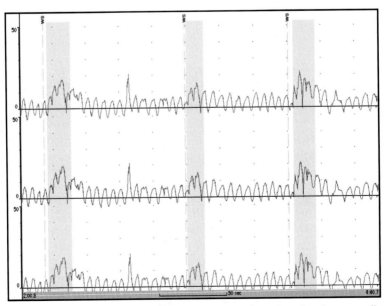

Figure 5-1. Portion of esophageal body tracing showing low amplitude peristaltic waves characteristic of poor contractility in "scleroderma like" esophagus. This would make me reconsider surgical intervention. Each vertical dashed line indicates a swallow.

the operation, I believe the performance of this procedure is mandatory preoperatively. Although the available data suggest that a Nissen fundoplication (360-degree fundoplication) is the operation of choice regardless of the preoperative motility findings, in the presence of a "scleroderma-like esophagus" (Figure 5-1), in which the amplitude of distal esophageal contractions is far below 20 mm Hg, the surgeon must take care and carefully consider whether to proceed as the operation may be more prone to failure or postoperative dysphagia. Although rare, there are patients referred to and sent for antireflux surgery who have achalasia that for whatever reason is missed preoperatively and when this happens, a 360-degree wrap would most certainly portend postoperative dysphagia. Unfortunately, our society remains litigious and if there is a preoperative motility abnormality, as noted above, that is not discovered, this may create problems in the postoperative period. Most importantly, in expert hands preoperative manometry can be performed in 15 to 30 minutes, a small "investment of time" to rule out potential risks for operative intervention. In addition, I always obtain a barium swallow prior to surgery so that the operating surgeon is aware of the size of the hiatal hernia and of esophageal length as this may alter their operative approach.

Bibliography

DeVault KR, Castell DO. American College of Gastroenterology. Updated guidelines for the diagnosis and treatment of gastroesophageal reflux disease. *Am J Gastroenterol.* 2005;100(1):190-200.

WHAT ARE THE INDICATIONS FOR 24-HOUR AMBULATORY pH MONITORING? WHICH OF MY PATIENTS SHOULD HAVE THIS STUDY "ON MEDICATIONS" VERSUS "OFF MEDICATIONS"?

Ambulatory pH monitoring or ambulatory reflux monitoring is the only means of documenting the presence of abnormal esophageal acid exposure and abnormal reflux frequency and to correlate the association of symptoms and reflux episodes. The most common indication for pH/reflux monitoring is evaluation of patients with symptoms suspected due to GERD who have not responded to proton pump inhibitors (PPIs). This is the only way to document the presence or absence of continued reflux, the association of reflux with symptoms, and to document adequacy of PPI therapy in acid control. As almost every patient has been on at least one PPI and often twice-daily therapy (many on H_2 receptor antagonists [H_2RAs] at bedtime), we are most often performing studies on therapy to determine if the continued symptoms are due to reflux. In many more cases, we are later also performing a study off therapy to determine if the original suspicion of GERD can be supported. If we perform a study off therapy, we discontinue PPIs for at least 7 days, though 10 days is ideal as one study has shown some efficacy in pH control for esomeprazole for 10 days after discontinuing the drug. Our off-therapy studies are almost exclusively done using 48-hour telemetry capsule monitoring (Bravo). This technology is more patient (and physician) friendly and offers the additional 24-hour monitoring (or longer) period. The most difficult decision revolves around the most efficacious method for on therapy pH monitoring. The Bravo capsule offers the convenience mentioned above and allows efficiency as it can be placed at the time of endoscopic evaluation (or transorally if the squamocolumnar line is known). One study improved detection of symptoms by having a 2nd day of monitoring and added sensitivity and specificity of symptom calculation. In our experience, discordance between day 1 and day 2 interpretation (normal day 1, abnormal day 2) is seen even when patients are on therapy, making overall interpretation somewhat complex. If Bravo is the only monitoring device available, the decision is easy; it should be placed at the time of endoscopy if it is nondiagnostic. In addition, the telemetry capsule is ideal for monitoring acid control in Barrett's patients; it gives reliable 48-hour data and in my experience can be attached in the columnar lining at any level above the top of the gastric folds. The limitation of the technique is the inability to monitor patients at multiple levels in the esophagus simultaneously (technical issues and costs), to perform intragastric pH monitoring, or to detect non-acid reflux. Monitoring at multiple levels and intragastric pH monitoring is of value in limited situations. Nonacid reflux requires impedance technology.

Many of the decisions regarding whether to perform pH monitoring on or off therapy or with Bravo or impedance/pH are individualized. Testing off therapy is used in my practice for patients in whom there is a low index of suspicion for reflux disease, to "rule out GERD" on the basis of quantitatively normal esophageal acid exposure. A negative pH study performed with the patient off PPI therapy is generally considered evidence that a patient does not have pathologic reflux disease, especially when combined with a negative symptom index. I utilize off-therapy pH testing to document GERD in patients without endoscopic esophagitis who are being evaluated for endoscopic antireflux therapy or fundoplication. The key to off-therapy pH testing is to demonstrate abnormal reflux and association between reflux and symptoms. Symptom-reflux correlation using the symptom index (SI) is useful but can be inaccurate. The symptom association probability (SAP) is a better statistical method but not as simple to use day to day.

I use on-therapy testing commonly to evaluate patients with refractory reflux symptoms. The goal is to determine if the patient is having persistently abnormal distal esophageal acid exposure in spite of PPI therapy and if symptoms are correlated. The likelihood of having an abnormal pH study on PPI therapy is variable, depends upon the clinical setting and indication for the test. On twice-daily PPI therapy, only 4% of patients had abnormal pH monitoring in one study. Patients with Barrett's, however, even if asymptomatic, will have reflux overnight in up to 50% even on twice-daily PPI. Others have found that over 20% of patients on PPI still have abnormal acid exposure. Even if the overall percentage of patients with persistent acid reflux on PPI therapy is small, I believe that pH monitoring is still of clinical utility to identify truly refractory patients who may benefit from additional medical, endoscopic, or surgical therapy. A limitation of on-therapy testing is that the reduction of gastric acid converts acid to weakly acid or non-acid reflux episodes that are not detected by pH monitoring. The clinical importance of "non-acid reflux" is a controversy best addressed through ongoing investigations using esophageal impedance monitoring.

More often I am evaluating patients on their current therapy to assess symptom association and efficacy of antisecretory therapy in control of pH and then subsequently performing pH monitoring OFF therapy to determine if reflux was present at baseline. This is increasingly necessary in patients with ENT-related complaints. These patients are given a diagnosis of laryngopharyngeal reflux and treated primarily based on ENT signs and symptoms. They are often on high doses of antisecretory therapy, have normal esophagoscopy, and have not had a diagnosis of gastroesophageal reflux disease confirmed. In this

Table 6-1

Recommendations for Ambulatory Esophageal pH, Impedance Monitoring, and Bile Acid Reflux Testing

pH Monitoring Is Useful

1. Document abnormal esophageal acid exposure in an endoscopy-negative patient being considered for endoscopic or surgical antireflux procedure. An abnormal pH study does not, however, causally link reflux with a specific presenting symptom. Use of symptom association analyses provide information in this regard but have not been adequately validated.
2. Evaluation of endoscopy-negative patients with typical reflux symptoms that are refractory to PPI therapy.
   a. pH study done on therapy but consider extended testing with wireless pH system incorporating periods of both off- and on-therapy testing. The diagnostic yield of on-therapy testing in patients who have not symptomatically responded to bid PPI therapy is limited.
   b. Use of a symptom correlation measure (SI, SSI, or SAP) is recommended to statistically interpret the causality of a particular symptom with episodes of acid reflux. Such measures can be applied even in the presence of esophageal acid exposure values that fall within the normal range. These statistical measures, however, do not ensure a response to either medical or surgical antireflux therapies. The yield of symptom association is increased when pH study is done for 48 hours and off PPI therapy compared with 24 hours and on PPI therapy, respectively.
   c. Routine proximal or intragastric pH monitoring not recommended.

pH Monitoring May Be Useful

1. Document adequacy of PPI therapy in esophageal acid control in patients with complications of reflux disease that include Barrett's esophagus. The threshold for adequate suppression of esophageal acid exposure on PPI therapy has not been defined. Furthermore, data supporting the clinical importance of achieving normalization of esophageal acid exposure in such patients are limited.
2. Evaluation of endoscopy-negative patients with atypical reflux symptoms that are refractory to bid PPI therapy. The diagnostic yield of pH testing under such circumstances is low.
   a. pH study done on bid PPI therapy in patients with high pretest probability of GERD or off therapy in patients with low pretest probability of GERD. Pretest probability is based on prevalence of GERD in patient population under question, clinician's impression, and degree of response to empiric PPI trial. Consider extended pH study to incorporate periods both off and on PPI therapy.
   b. Use of symptom correlation recommended for selected symptoms that include chest pain. Use of symptom correlation in the evaluation of chronic laryngeal symptoms, asthma, and cough is of unproven benefit.
   c. Routine proximal or intragastric pH monitoring not recommended.

(continued)

case we use the 48-hour Bravo capsule for testing. Ultimately, a thorough evaluation of the GERD patient may require impedance/pH monitoring on therapy and 48-hour Bravo off therapy to satisfy the patient and referring physician as to the diagnosis.

The latest guidelines for performance of ambulatory pH monitoring are indicated in Table 6-1.

<u>Table 6-1</u> *(continued)*

Recommendations for Ambulatory Esophageal pH, Impedance Monitoring, and Bile Acid Reflux Testing

Combined pH Monitoring with Esophageal Impedance Monitoring May Be Useful

1. Evaluation of endoscopy-negative patients with complaints of heartburn or regurgitation despite PPI therapy in whom documentation of non-acid reflux will alter clinical management. The increased diagnostic yield of impedance monitoring over conventional pH monitoring for symptom association is highest when performed on PPI therapy and nominal off PPI therapy.
2. Utility of impedance monitoring in refractory reflux patients with primary complaints of chest pain or extraesophageal symptoms is unproven.
3. Current interpretation of impedance monitoring relies on use of symptom correlation measures (SI, SSI, or SAP). The therapeutic implications of an abnormal impedance test are unproven at this time.

Bile Acid Reflux Testing May Be Useful

1. Evaluation of patients with persistent typical reflux symptoms in spite of demonstrated normalization of distal esophageal acid exposure by pH study. Impedance monitoring may obviate the need for bile acid reflux testing under such circumstances.
2. Bile acid reflux testing equipment currently has very limited commercial availability.

Reprinted from Hirano I, Richter JE, and the Practice Parameters Committee of the American College of Gastroenterology. Esophageal reflux testing. *Am J Gastroenterol.* 2007;102(3):668-685, with permission from Elsevier.

Bibliography

Charbel S, Khandwala F, Vaezi MF. The role of esophageal pH monitoring in symptomatic patients on PPI therapy. *Am J Gastroenterol.* 2005;100:283-289.

DeVault KR, Castell DO. Updated guidelines for the diagnosis and treatment of gastroesophageal reflux disease. The Practice Parameters Committee of the American College of Gastroenterology. *Am J Gastroenterol.* 1999;94:1434-1442.

Hirano I, Richter JE, and the Practice Parameters Committee of the American College of Gastroenterology. Esophageal reflux testing. *Am J Gastroenterol.* 2007;102(3):668-685.

Kahrilas PJ, Quigley EM. Clinical esophageal pH recording: a technical review for practice guideline development. *Gastroenterology.* 1996;110:1982-1996.

Mikles D, Gerson LB, Triadafilopoulos G. Complete elimination of reflux symptoms does not guarantee normalization of intraesophageal and intragastric pH in patients with gastroesophageal reflux disease (GERD). *Am J Gastroenterol.* 2004;99:991-996.

MY PATIENT HAS DYSPHONIA THAT I BELIEVE IS DUE TO REFLUX, BUT HER 24-HOUR pH PROBE ON BID PANTOPRAZOLE WAS NEGATIVE. ARE THERE OTHER REFLUX TESTS THAT I SHOULD CONSIDER?

Patients with symptoms suspected due to GERD who are refractory to antisecretory therapy fall into the following categories: (1) GERD is the correct diagnosis and the patient is suboptimally treated for acid reflux. This is a patient with an extraesophageal or atypical symptom suspected due to GERD. In this case antisecretory therapy can be optimized in the short or long term and/or the patient offered endoscopic or antireflux surgery. (2) The patient has non-acid reflux. Early impedance/pH studies suggest this is seen in a small but important minority, most often with typical symptoms of regurgitation and heartburn. What is not clear is whether the symptoms are produced by abnormal frequency or volume of reflux or hypersensitivity to physiologic amounts. This area is clearly in evolution. (3) The diagnosis of GERD is incorrect. Either the patient has residual symptoms neither related to acid or non-acid reflux *or* the patient did not have GERD in the first place. The latter is seen with increasing frequency as higher doses of antisecretory therapy are given empirically. Although this practice in many cases is reasonable, it may complicate evaluation later. The evaluation of these patients requires a full evaluation including careful review of the history, compliance with therapy, upper gastrointestinal endoscopy, and prolonged reflux monitoring, often both on and off antisecretory therapy.

There are little data on the incidence or prevalence of continued laryngeal symptoms in patients treated with higher doses of proton pump inhibitors either given once or twice daily. Therefore, in developing an approach to these patients, one must use indirect data from pH monitoring studies performed in patients (subjects) on proton pump inhibitors (PPIs) either once or twice daily. These studies have made us well aware of the prevalence of what has been termed nocturnal gastric acid breakthrough, a pharmacodynamic phenomenon in which 70% to 80% of patients taking proton pump inhibitors twice daily will have periods of intragastric pH falling to below 4 for greater than 60 minutes in the overnight period. What is less frequently discussed is the prevalence of continued esophageal acid exposure in this patient population. Some esophageal acid exposure is seen in 15% of patients with GERD (without Barrett's esophagus) studied with combined intraesophageal and intragastric pH monitoring on twice-daily PPI. Almost 10% of patients on twice-daily proton pump inhibitors who complain of continued heartburn have some esophageal acid exposure that is associated with symptoms. Thus a small number of patients with continued heartburn respond to even higher doses of antisecretory therapy. In contrast, few patients with abnormal esophageal acid exposure and little response to increase in antisecretory therapy in patients with extraesophageal GERD symptoms. A review of our own database (>400 studies on bid PPI) supports these data. Patients with *heartburn* and *regurgitation* are more likely to have continued acid reflux compared to extraesophageal symptoms. In further support of a small but potential treatable number with continued acid exposure on high-dose PPI are preliminary results of studies evaluating the efficacy of combined impedance/pH studies in work up of "refractory patients." Two have found that just under 10% will have symptoms associated with continued acid reflux. A body of literature has documented continued esophageal acid exposure (particularly at night) in patients with Barrett's esophagus, despite treatment with twice-daily PPI. Several studies reveal that a substantial number will have abnormal esophageal reflux despite being asymptomatic. Although there are no definitive data available that support treating this continued asymptomatic reflux, accumulating intermediate marker data and a retrospective case review showing a decrease in dysplasia in patients on PPIs compared to those on H_2 receptor antagonists (H$_2$RAs) or no therapy have led this author further toward strong support of aggressive management. No definitive studies have documented continued reflux as the cause of refractory strictures; however, there are studies showing incomplete response to 40 mg omeprazole and most of us have seen a refractory stricture that responded to higher doses of PPI or antireflux surgery.

The recent availability of multichannel intraluminal impedance monitoring has made it possible to detect reflux events in which the esophageal pH does not drop <4. This so-called non-acid (weakly acidic) reflux appears to be associated with some symptoms, though definitive outcome studies remain to be performed. Early results support that if any symptom is likely to be "truly" associated with a non-acid reflux event it is *regurgitation*, with heartburn the second most likely. Again extraesophageal symptoms appear less likely to be associated. The most recent American College of Gastroenterology (ACG) guidelines suggest that combined impedance/pH monitoring may be useful. I would perform impedance testing in my practice.

The optimal approach to the patient with typical or atypical symptoms suspected due to GERD who is still symptomatic on twice-daily PPI is to perform a thorough and careful evaluation to determine if reflux is responsible. This often involves multiple interventions,

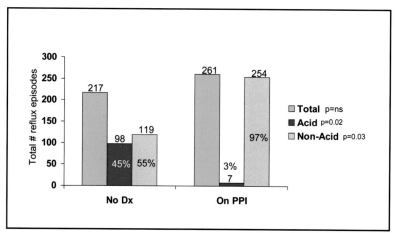

Figure 7-1. (Reprinted from Vela MF, Camacho-Lobato L, Srinivasan R, Tutuian R, Katz PO, Castell DO. Simultaneous intraesophageal impedance and pH measurement of acid and non-acid gastroesophageal reflux: effect of omeprazole. *Gastroenterology.* 2001;120:1599-1606, with permission from Elsevier.)

including determining whether the patient had GERD in the first place. In our practice the evaluation includes a careful history of PPI compliance and dose timing. Despite continued teaching of the importance of dosing PPIs prior to a meal, this is often ignored. When omeprazole IR is prescribed, many completely disregard meal timing. Although bedtime administration of this drug is reasonable it is not clear that it can be taken anytime of day. I do not advocate the empiric use of H_2RA at bedtime, nor addition of a prokinetic agent unless nocturnal reflux and/or erosive esophagitis has been documented. In my experience the overall likelihood of success is low when H_2RA is used empirically, and prolonged pH more valuable. We perform endoscopy if one has not been done or carefully reported. This is granted of low yield from the standpoint of finding erosive esophagitis but may document the presence of Barrett's, a rare but other structural cause for symptoms (large hernia, ulcer), and allows for accurate placement of a telemetry pH capsule. In addition, there is the still to be defined value of a negative endoscopy for the patient and indeed the treating physician. Barium studies are rarely performed except in the presence of dysphagia, in which case we would suspect achalasia (Figure 7-1).

Bibliography

Katz PO. GERD symptoms on antisecretory therapy: acid, non-acid or no GERD. *Rev Gastroenterol Disord.* 2006;6(3):136-145.

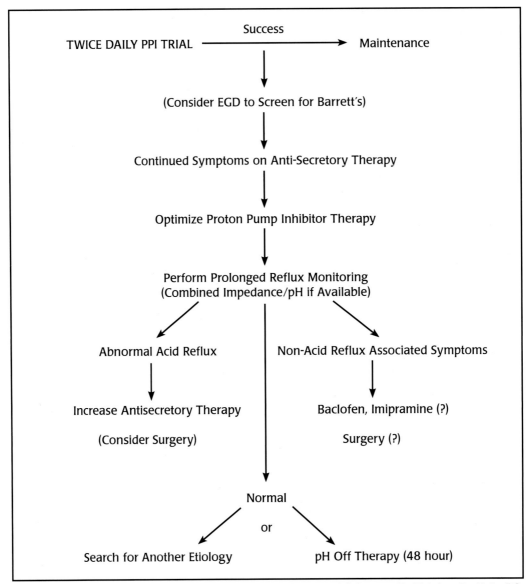

Figure 7-2. (Reprinted from Vela MF, Camacho-Lobato L, Srinivasan R, Tutuian R, Katz PO, Castell DO. Simultaneous intraesophageal impedance and pH measurement of acid and non-acid gastroesophageal reflux: effect of omeprazole. *Gastroenterology*. 2001;120:1599-1606, with permission from Elsevier.)

MR. JONES HAS CLASSIC REFLUX SYMPTOMS EVEN WHILE TAKING BID ESOMEPRAZOLE. I HAVE CONSIDERED A pH PROBE WITH IMPEDANCE TO DOCUMENT NON-ACID REFLUX, BUT I AM WONDERING WHAT THERAPY I CAN PROVIDE EVEN IF THIS TEST IS CONCLUSIVE?

The availability of combined multichannel intraluminal impedance (MII) pH monitoring has added to our ability to evaluate patients with symptoms suspected due to GERD refractory to antisecretory therapy. This technology allows the assessment of both acid (pH) and non-acid (impedance) reflux. A series of studies with this technology evaluating patients with symptoms suggestive of reflux on proton pump inhibitor therapy have documented the presence of non-acid reflux and their association with symptoms. Thus if in the judgment of the clinician, the patient has symptoms caused by non-acid reflux, decisions regarding therapy are complex as few controlled observations are available. "Reflux reduction" can be accomplished with a Nissen fundoplication, endoscopic therapy, lifestyle modifications, and so-called medical therapy. The latter conceptually include

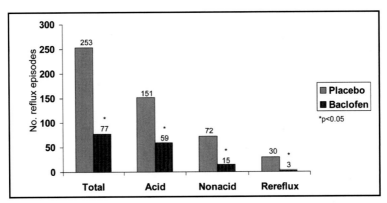

Figure 8-1. Effect of baclofen on acid and non-acid reflux. (Reprinted from Vela MF, Tutuian R, Katz PO, Castell DO. Baclofen decreases acid and non-acid post-prandial gastroesophageal reflux measured by combined multichannel intraluminal impedance and pH. *Aliment Pharmacol Ther.* 2003;17:243-251, with permission from Blackwell Scientific Publications.)

therapies that decrease transient lower esophageal sphincter relaxations, increase lower esophageal sphincter pressure, improve gastric emptying, decrease visceral sensation, and/or reflux. The best-studied "medical therapy" for consideration in patients with non-acid reflux is baclofen. This γ-aminobutyric acid (GABA) agonist has been shown in the laboratory to decrease the number of transient lower esophageal sphincter relaxations, predominantly in the postprandial period. In addition, the drug has been shown in the short term to decrease postprandial reflux of both acid and non-acid variety and has been demonstrated to have the potential to reduce symptoms as well (Figure 8-1). There are no clear dose recommendations for baclofen for use in non-acid reflux. When I use it (principally for patients with regurgitation as the primary symptom), I begin with a low dose, 5 mg either at bedtime or 3 times a day depending upon symptom frequency, and increase gradually to 10 mg 3 times daily. The drug is limited by side effects so that long-term use has been difficult in my limited experience. If the patient responds, then I would consider a fundoplication. One observational series has shown that laparoscopic Nissen fundoplication can offer a positive outcome in patients with non-acid reflux. It is my clinical impression that surgery is most valuable for patients with regurgitation and possibly for cough. The readers should be clear that fundoplication is not recommended in patients with symptoms refractory to proton pump inhibitor (PPI) unless a strong association with symptoms and non-acid reflux can be documented. This is particularly true in patients with laryngeal symptoms, who do not appear to respond to surgery if they have failed PPI.

In my practice I would routinely perform impedance/pH testing in this patient for the following reasons. If continued acid reflux is demonstrated, antisecretory therapy can be changed, reassessed, or increased. Surgery can be considered, though I rarely do this until after a new/different medical therapy trial. If non-acid reflux is found associated with symptoms, the patient can be offered an explanation for continued symptoms and possible therapy. If no association of symptoms and reflux are seen, acid control is optimal, and non-acid reflux frequency is normal (my findings in about 70% tested), then I can confidently say that reflux is not the cause of the symptoms recorded on the test tracing. Patient and referring physician can be reassured.

The most recent American College of Gastroenterology (ACG) guidelines offer suggestions about pH/impedance testing (see Question 6).

Bibliography

Hirano I, Richter JE, and the Practice Parameters Committee of the American College of Gastroenterology. Esophageal reflux testing. *Am J Gastroenterol.* 2007;102(3):668-685.

Tutuian R, Mainie I, Agrawal A, et al. Nonacid reflux in patients with chronic cough on acid-suppressive therapy. *Chest.* 2006;130(2):386-391.

WHAT IS THE ROLE OF DIETARY MODIFICATION IN THE MANAGEMENT OF PATIENTS WITH REFLUX?

Throughout "history" many have felt that GERD is a lifestyle disease under patients' control. As such, numerous dietary and lifestyle modifications continue to be advocated as important in therapy of GERD and sometimes aggressively "pushed" on patients (Table 9-1). Lifestyle and dietary modifications are based on physiologic data that certain foods, body positions, tobacco, alcohol, and body mass index (BMI) contribute to an increase in transient lower esophageal sphincter relaxations, reflux, or both. In addition, certain drugs have been documented to decrease lower esophageal sphincter pressure and have the potential to exacerbate reflux (Table 9-2). Other medications may cause direct esophageal injury and may exacerbate reflux symptoms. These include aspirin, nonaspirin, nonsteroidal anti-inflammatory drugs, some antibiotics, potassium chloride tablets, ferrous sulfate tablets, alendronate, and other bisphosphonates. Regardless of how sound the intent and the solid laboratory research, there are little outcome data to support aggressively pushing lifestyles to reluctant patients (Table 9-3). Recent data find limited support for the effectiveness of any lifestyle intervention on symptom relief. Despite this, guidelines from the American College of Gastroenterology continue to recommend lifestyle changes as adjuncts to pharmacologic treatment. It is my experience that most patients have already attempted their own lifestyle changes based on their own evidence of which dietary indiscretions and lifestyle issues exacerbate their disease.

Physicians sometimes make different recommendations for lifestyle modifications in different patient populations. Patients with newly diagnosed GERD were asked questions about 7 common lifestyle modifications physicians could have recommended. For 5 of these modifications, less than 50% of patients reported their health care providers had recommended them. Physicians are most likely to recommend lifestyle changes in patients less than 60 years of age than in older patients ($P = 0.002$); those who had a BMI over 30 kg/m^2 also received advice on eating habits more often than did other patients

Table 9-1
Traditional Lifestyle Modifications Indicated for Patients With GERD

Sleep	• Elevate head 6 inches • Sleep on left side • Wait at least 2 to 3 hours after eating before retiring
Diet	• Avoid such irritants as citrus, tomatoes, coffee, cola, alcohol, chocolate, peppermint • Eat less fat and more protein • Eat smaller meals
Smoking	• Decrease or stop
Medications to avoid	• Anticholinergics • Sedatives/tranquilizers • Theophylline • Prostaglandins • Calcium channel blockers • Alendronate
Other modifications	• Avoid tight clothing • Avoid straining to lift heavy objects • Avoid exercise after meals

Table 9-2
Medications That Can Decrease LESP

• Theophylline	• Nitrates
• Nifedipine	• Meperidine
• Anticholinergics	• Diazepam
• Prostaglandins	• Morphine
• Calcium channel blockers	• Anesthetic agents
• Alendronate	• α-Adrenergic antagonists
• Dopamine	• Oral β2-adrenergic agents
• Oral contraceptives	

($P = 0.047$). People who were heavy smokers were more likely to receive recommendations than people who were light smokers ($P = 0.001$). Lifestyle changes to counter GERD symptoms are rather precise, involving specific foods, beverages, and sleeping positions. For many patients, changing their diet by giving up orange juice, coffee, carbonated beverages,

Table 9-3

Recommendations Based on Results of a Review of Studies Involving Lifestyle Modifications

Lifestyle modification	Strength of scientific evidence	Pathophysiologically conclusive?	Recommendable?
Avoid fatty meals	Equivocal	Equivocal	Not generally
Avoid carbonated beverages	Moderate	Yes	Yes
Select decaffeinated beverages	Equivocal	Equivocal	Not generally
Avoid citrus	Weak	Yes	Not generally
Eat smaller meals	Weak	Yes	Yes
Lose weight	Equivocal	Equivocal	Yes*
Avoid alcoholic beverages	Weak	Mechanisms not understood; different alcoholic beverages have different effects	Not generally
Stop smoking	Weak	Yes	Yes (in symptomatic persons)
Avoid excessive exercise	Weak	Yes	Yes*
Sleep with head elevated	Equivocal	Equivocal	Not generally
Sleep on left side	Unequivocal	Yes	Yes

*Obesity and smoking appear to be risk factors for cancer of the distal esophagus.

and chocolate, for example, represents a serious impairment of their perceived quality of life. Many of these changes are a poor reflection of evidence-based medicine, because studies to prove benefits have produced contradictory results and have been conducted in small, often healthy populations. Some changes such as smoking cessation and weight reduction in patients who are obese carry well-accepted health benefits. Other changes may be less beneficial when measured against their cost in quality of life.

Bibliography

Hila A, Castell DO. Nighttime reflux is primarily an early event. *J Clin Gastroenterol.* 2005;39:579-583.

ARE ANY SPECIFIC LIFESTYLE CHANGES BETTER THAN OTHERS?

Multiple dietary and lifestyle modifications continue to be advocated in therapy of GERD. Lifestyle and dietary modifications are based on physiologic data that certain foods, body positions, tobacco, alcohol, and body mass index contribute to an increase in transient lower esophageal sphincter relaxations, reflux, or both. In addition, certain drugs have been documented to decrease lower esophageal sphincter pressure and have the potential to exacerbate reflux. Other medications such as aspirin, nonaspirin, non-steroidal anti-inflammatory drugs, some antibiotics, potassium chloride tablets, ferrous sulfate tablets, alendronate, and other bisphosphonates may cause direct esophageal injury and may exacerbate reflux symptoms. There are little data to support the effectiveness of any lifestyle intervention on symptom relief. However, American College of Gastroenterology guidelines continue to recommend lifestyle changes as adjuncts to pharmacologic treatment. It is my experience that most patients have already attempted their own lifestyle changes based on their own evidence of which dietary indiscretions and lifestyle issues exacerbate their disease.

Of all the recommendations, reminding and encouraging patients to avoid going to bed with a full stomach is the most logical. Proximal acid migration is greatest during sleep and sleep delays esophageal acid clearance (Figures 10-1 and 10-2). This is supported by a recent study showing that most reflux occurs in the first 4 hours of the sleeping period and that patients eating with 2 hours of sleep were 2.5 times more likely to have abnormal nocturnal reflux (Figure 10-3). This observation is not the only one of its kind. I see many who are helped with nocturnal symptoms if they can avoid a big meal, late at night.

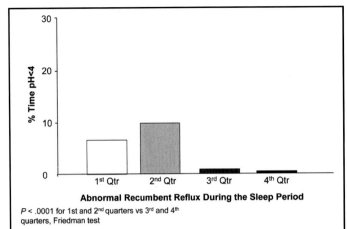

Figure 10-1. Effect of sleep on esophageal acid clearance time. A small study showing that acid infused in the distal esophagus is cleared more rapidly when the patient is awake than asleep. (Reprinted from Hila A, Castell DO. Nighttime reflux is primarily an early event. *J Clin Gastroenterol.* 2005;39[7]:579-583, with permission from Raven Press.)

Bibliography

Kaltenbach T, Crockett S, Gerson LB. Are lifestyle measures effective in patients with gastroesophageal reflux disease? An evidence-based approach. *Arch Intern Med.* 2006;166(9):965-971.

Kinoshita Y. Review article: treatment for gastro-oesophageal reflux disease—lifestyle advice and mediaction. *Aliment Pharmacol Ther.* 2004;20(Suppl 8):19-23.

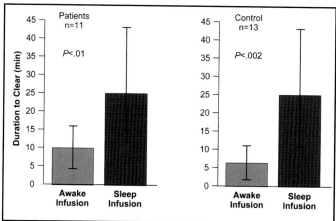

Figure 10-2. Proximal migration of esophageal acid perfusions during waking and sleep. Similar methodology to Figure 10-1 revealing that distal esophageal acid infusion is likely to be cleared rapidly when awake and supine and propagated proximally when asleep. (Reprinted from Orr WC, Robinson MG, Johnson LF. Acid clearance during sleep in the pathogenesis of reflux esophagitis. *Dig Dis Sci.* 1981;26:423-427, with permission from Springer Science and Business Media.)

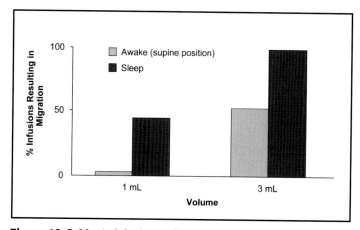

Figure 10-3. Most nighttime reflux occurs in the first half of sleep. Study reviewed pH tracings of patients studied off treatment, divided sleeping period into quartile, and demonstrated high frequency of reflux early in sleeping period. The implications for therapy are real. An empty stomach will help. In addition, a delayed-release proton pump inhibitor given before dinner should control pH into the critical sleeping period. Alternatively, omeprazole immediate release may be dosed at bedtime as an alternative strategy. I find some patients who do well with once-daily dosing before dinner, including management of daytime symptoms. (Reprinted from Orr WC, Eisenbruch S, Harnish MJ, Johnson LF. Proximal migration of esophageal acid perfusions during waking and sleeping. *Am J Gastroenterol.* 2000;95:37-42, with permission from Elsevier.)

WHAT IS THE OPTIMAL USE OF OVER-THE-COUNTER ANTACIDS AND H_2 RECEPTOR ANTAGONISTS IN THE MANAGEMENT OF REFLUX PATIENTS?

Antacids are the most widely used agents for treating GERD because patients with mild heartburn often self-medicate with these over-the-counter drugs and never seek treatment for their reflux symptoms. Available in liquid and tablet forms, antacids are used as needed. Some patients use antacids to supplement other anti-GERD therapies. In clinical practice, antacids help to control mild-to-moderate reflux symptoms in a large proportion of patients. Because they act locally, antacids are considered first-line therapy for pregnant women who experience heartburn. However, magnesium-containing agents should be avoided in the latter part of pregnancy.

Alginic acid is often given in combination with an antacid. The first component provides a floating barrier on the gastric pool to minimize the contact between gastric contents and esophageal mucosa, whereas the antacid temporarily neutralizes stomach acid. As with antacids alone, in clinical practice, this combination therapy helps control mild-to-moderate reflux symptoms. Improvement in GERD symptoms occurred in 3 of 4 studies that compared alginate/antacid combination therapy with placebo. However, when compared with antacids, the alginate combination therapy was superior in only 1 of 4 studies. Convincing proof of esophageal healing has never been obtained in any study, and alginic acid therapy is probably no better than antacid therapy in treating moderate-to-severe GERD.

Antacids and alginic acid are more effective than placebo in the relief of heartburn and combined antacid and alginic acid therapy may be superior to antacids alone in the control of symptoms. In high doses, antacids are no more effective in healing erosive esophagitis than placebo and are most effective when given in the first hour after a meal. Of the multiple agents on the market, there is no evidence that one antacid is better than the other. My experience is that many patients will use antacids to supplement prescription antisecretory therapy. Little evidence is available to support this and I find these agents of little value in my practice outside of the pregnant patient.

H_2 Receptor Antagonists

The 4 available agents, cimetidine, ranitidine, famotidine, and nizatidine, derive their efficacy in GERD exclusively by inhibition of acid secretion. H_2 receptor antagonists (H_2RAs) only block 1 receptor, thus have limited effect on acid reduction and are relatively weak inhibitors of meal-stimulated acid secretion. The antisecretory capabilities of H_2RAs are best at night, with duration of acid inhibition longer when the drug is taken in the evening or before bedtime. Equipotent doses of H_2RAs equally inhibit acid secretion, thus similar efficacy in GERD. H_2RAs were made available as over the counter agents in 1995 and are now available in half- and full-strength doses. Combination therapy with H_2RA/antacids are available over the counter.

Despite multiple studies showing inferior pH control, symptom relief and healing of erosive esophagitis compared to proton pump inhibitors, standard dose H_2RAs are still recommended as the first choice for treatment in many step-up algorithms, usually for reasons of cost. Although the upfront costs may be lower, in 2007 patient expectations for adequate symptom relief are rarely met by continuous H_2RAs. Whether because of the development of tolerance or plain superiority of proton pump inhibitors (PPIs), it is difficult to recommend H_2RAs as primary therapy for GERD.

Combination H_2RA and PPI

Adding an H_2 blocker at bedtime to PPI therapy to control nighttime symptoms has been popular since the late 1990s when pharmacodynamic studies demonstrated short-term efficacy in control of nocturnal pH when used in this manner. Tachyphylaxis with long-term use has been demonstrated which limits the efficacy of these agents when used daily.

A series of pharmacodynamic studies shows a hierarchy of pH control starting with a PPI before breakfast, adding an H_2RA at bedtime, increasing to twice-daily PPI monotherapy, and finally adding an H_2RA at bedtime to twice-daily PPI therapy. No clinical trials demonstrate any symptom improvement with any of these regimens over a PPI alone, so it likely would be most practical to add an H_2RA at bedtime to PPI therapy on an as-needed basis for reasons of cost (Table 11-1).

In my current practice, H_2RAs are most useful for prevention of provocable nighttime breakthrough symptoms in patients already on high-dose PPIs. This method may decrease tachyphylaxis and offers patients flexibility in dosing if breakthrough symptoms are infrequent. Otherwise, I do not use H_2RAs.

Table 11-1

Hierarchy

- PPI once a day
- PPI plus H_2 HS (OTC probably OK)*
- PPI bid*
- PPI bid plus H_2* or esomeprazole bid*

*These regimens have never been tested head to head in clinical trials!

Bibliography

Fackler WK, Ours TM, Vaezi MF, Richter JE. Long-term effect of H_2RA therapy on nocturnal gastric acid breakthrough. *Gastroenterology.* 2002;122(3):625-632.

Peghini PL, Katz PO, Castell DO. Ranitidine controls nocturnal gastric acid breakthrough on omeprazole: a controlled study in normal subjects. *Gastroenterology.* 1998;115:1335-1339.

DR. SMITH SUGGESTED THAT I ADD RANITIDINE 150 MG AT BEDTIME TO A REGIMEN OF BID ESOMEPRAZOLE. IS THERE ANY EVIDENCE THAT THIS HELPS PATIENTS WITH SYMPTOMS OF GERD?

The use of H_2 receptor antagonists (H_2RAs) given at bedtime in addition to twice-daily proton pump inhibitor (PPI) was popularized in the late 1990s after a publication demonstrating that the overnight recovery of gastric acid secretion seen in patients on twice-daily proton pump inhibitors could be reduced to a greater extent with a bedtime dose of ranitidine 150 or 300 mg compared to an additional dose of a proton pump inhibitor at bedtime. The maximal effect on overnight pH is with the first dose, with a decrease in efficacy in pH control over time (tachyphylaxis) (Figure 12-1). The key to decisions regarding the addition of an H_2 antagonist in this patient are based on review of 2 studies.

A prospective study (Figure 12-2) of 23 normal volunteers and 20 GERD patients were studied at baseline with omeprazole 20 mg bid (before breakfast and dinner) for 2 weeks followed by the addition of an H_2 receptor antagonist (ranitidine 300 mg qhs) at bedtime for 28 days. Patients were studied with prolonged ambulatory pH monitoring after days 1, 7, and 28 of continuous H_2 receptor antagonists at bedtime. The median time pH < 4 for overnight period was similar between patients and volunteers so were considered together. Four patterns of gastric pH response were found: The first group experienced a decreasing effect of baseline H_2RA over time (tolerance). The second consisted of 21% who exhibited a sustained response to H_2RA therapy (no tolerance). The third group had no acid recovery on PPI twice daily and remained so when H_2RA was added. All in this group were *Helicobacter pylori* positive. The fourth group was marked by an unpredictable response (26%). This group showed variable outcome at different time points in their study.

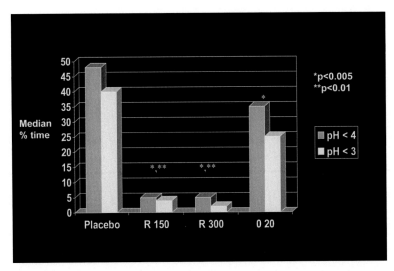

Figure 12-1. Nocturnal acid breakthrough on bid PPIs. Effect of an H₂RA or PPI at bedtime. A study in which normal subjects were given omeprazole 20 mg twice daily for 1 week, followed by a single dose of ranitidine 150 mg, 300 mg, placebo, and omeprazole 20 mg at bedtime in random order, shows that a single dose of H₂RA at bedtime is best at reducing overnight acid. (Reprinted from Peghini PL, Katz PO, Castell DO. Ranitidine controls nocturnal gastric acid breakthrough on omeprazole: a controlled study in normal subjects. *Gastroenterology.* 1998;115:1335-1339, with permission from Elsevier.)

Another retrospective study (Figure 12-3) reviewed prolonged ambulatory pH monitoring studies in patients comprised of 3 groups. Group 1 = 60 patients taking either omeprazole 20 mg or lansoprazole 30 mg twice a day. Group 2 = 45 patients on proton pump inhibitor twice a day (omeprazole 20 mg or lansoprazole 30 mg) plus an H₂ blocker at bedtime (ranitidine 300 mg, famotidine 40 mg, or nizatidine 300 mg) for greater than 28 days. Group 3 = 11 patients who were evaluated with both regimens. Twenty-seven percent of patients spent 100% of the recumbent period with intragastric pH greater than 4, 32% with greater than 90% of recumbent period above 4 with the remainder scattered at varying degrees. This was superior to PPI bid ($P < 0.001$). For patients tested on both regimens ($n = 11$), median percentage time intragastric pH > 4 overnight increased from 54.6% without H₂RA to 96.5% with H₂RA hs ($P = 0.001$).

These studies come to different conclusions; the former that there is no sustained control of intragastric pH over time with the addition of an H₂RA (i.e., tolerance develops), and the latter that there is substantial benefit to the long-term use of these agents at bedtime. Careful evaluation of these studies suggest many similarities. In the prospective study, 21% had a sustained response remarkably similar to the 27% in the retrospective study. The absence of statistical improvement in the prospective study ($P = 0.06$ at 1 week, $P = 0.08$ at 1 month) may represent a type II error. Both identify a substantial number of patients who have a sustained effect and many who do not. Both agree that achieving total acid control (100% time intragastric pH is > 4) is extremely difficult.

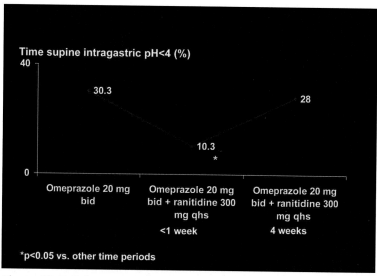

Figure 12-2. Tolerance to single doses of H_2RA as add-on therapy to PPI bid. This study shows overall no advantage to H_2RA long term when a group of subjects is studied and reminds the clinician to individualize the use of H_2RA. (Reprinted from Fackler WK, Ours TM, Vaezi MF, Richter JE. Long-term effect of H_2RA therapy on nocturnal gastric acid breakthrough. *Gastroenterology.* 2002;122[3]:625-632, with permission from Elsevier.)

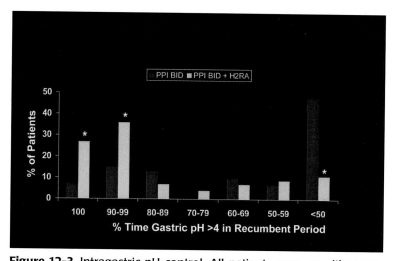

Figure 12-3. Intragastric pH control. All patients were on either proton pump inhibitor twice daily or twice daily plus H_2RA at bedtime for more than 28 days. Intragastric pH control is variable but overall superior with night time H_2RA.

Fortunately, this degree of pharmacologic control is rarely necessary. It is reasonable to conclude that tolerance to H_2RAs at bedtime is real but relative and that a sustained response may be seen in some patients. Unfortunately, there are no prospective symptom studies that allow us to answer the question raised here. The practical approach to the patient with refractory symptoms on twice-daily PPI is to study them and if acid reflux remains overnight, an H_2RA can be considered. In my practice, I use H_2RAs at bedtime less frequently because the availability of immediate-release omeprazole sodium bicarbonate. I find H_2RAs most efficacious when used on demand to prevent heartburn at night for patients with heartburn that is provoked for example by a late meal or a large meal at night. (See Figure 12-3 for an additional study on tolerance.)

Bibliography

Fackler WK, Ours TM, Vaezi MF, Richter JE. Long-term effect of H_2RA therapy on nocturnal gastric acid breakthrough. *Gastroenterology*. 2002;122(3):625-632.

Xue S, Katz PO, Banerjee P, Tutuian R, Castell DO. Bedtime H_2 blockers improve nocturnal gastric acid control in GERD patients on proton pump inhibitors. Aliment Pharmacol Ther. 2001;15:1351-1356.

IS AN EMPIRIC TRIAL OF PPI THERAPY EFFICACIOUS IN PATIENTS WITH SUSPECTED GERD? IN WHAT CIRCUMSTANCES?

The initial management of patients with symptoms suspected due to gastroesophageal reflux disease remains controversial. No single approach has diagnostic or therapeutic certainty. Early endoscopy lacks sensitivity for erosive esophagitis—up to 50% or greater will have normal mucosa on traditional endoscopy. Recent studies suggest that microscopic changes can be found in patients with heartburn and a normal endoscopy, suggesting there is a continuum from microscopic to macroscopic disease in some patients. Unfortunately, light microscopy does not reliably identify these changes and universal pathologic agreement and skill does not exist. As such, early endoscopy is not a reliable differentiation of who has GERD and who does not. In addition, it is impractical and indeed expensive to evaluate all patients with heartburn and/or dyspepsia (much less extraesophageal symptoms) prior to initiating treatment. Other studies such as barium swallow and prolonged ambulatory pH (reflux) monitoring have problems with sensitivity, specificity, and patient acceptance so it is difficult to argue that any test is a true gold standard for GERD.

As such, management has evolved to accept that symptom resolution with antisecretory therapy is the final arbiter of whether acid reflux is the ultimate cause for symptoms. Thus most experts and guideline documents and support or recommend a trial of empiric therapy in patients with uncomplicated presentations.

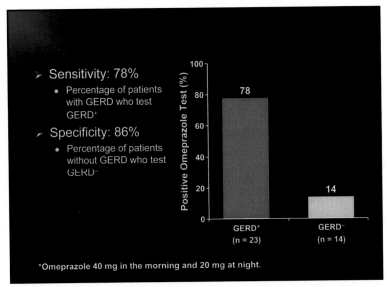

Figure 13-1. PPI test for GERD-associated noncardiac chest pain. In this study, patients were evaluated for reflux with endoscopy and pH monitoring. GERD (+) if abnormal endoscopy or pH. GERD (−) if both normal. A 1-week PPI test demonstrated good sensitivity and better specificity in these patients as diagnostic tests for GERD. (Reprinted from Fass R, Fennerty MB, Ofman JJ, et al. The clinical and economic value of a short course of omeprazole in patients with noncardiac chest pain. *Gastroenterology*. 1998;115[1]:42-49, with permission from Elsevier.)

So a patient who presents with classic heartburn and/or dyspepsia, with or without regurgitation, who has no dysphagia, odynophagia, bleeding, or other suspicion for a complicated disease can be treated with empiric therapy. Patients with other so-called atypical presentations of gastroesophageal reflux disease are equally controversial. Patients with noncardiac chest pain, for example, may have multiple etiologies—GERD, motility abnormalities, or so-called sensitive or irritable esophagus. Distinguishing among these is difficult using endoscopy, pH testing, or manometry. Endoscopy is abnormal less than 35% of the time and the presence of erosive esophagitis does not guarantee that GERD is the cause of the chest pain. pH testing reveals abnormal esophageal acid exposure in about 50%, with a slight increase if a symptom index is calculated but also does not make certain GERD is causative. Few patients have chest pain during a manometry study and GERD cannot be ruled out by this approach. As such, a therapeutic (empiric) antisecretory trial has been studied and found to be the most efficient and perhaps cost effective (Figure 13-1). It is now standard of practice.

The prevalence of GERD in patients with cough, asthma, laryngitis, erosion of dental enamel, and other non-heartburn presentations of reflux disease is variable, depending upon symptoms and the study. As the causes for these symptoms are multifactorial, GERD may be the cause or in fact simply be a cofactor and the patient have 2 diseases. Neither endoscopy nor pH monitoring is predictive of response of extraesophageal symptoms. As such, again, the response to antisecretory therapy becomes even more an arbiter

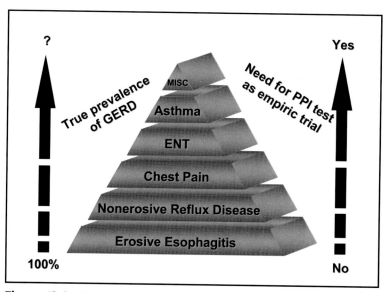

Figure 13-2. The Acid Reflux Pyramid. The pyramid illustrates the "certainty of GERD" balanced against the need for a proton pump inhibitor (PPI) trial.

of success as outlined in Figure 13-2. Empiric therapy is thus the approach of choice across most symptom presentations provided there is no suspicion of complication.

Bibliography

DeVault KR, Castell DO. American College of Gastroenterology. Updated guidelines for the diagnosis and treatment of gastroesophageal reflux disease. *Am J Gastroenterol.* 2005; 100(1):190-200.

Fass R, Fennerty MB, Ofman JJ, et al. The clinical and economic value of a short course of omeprazole in patients with noncardiac chest pain. *Gastroenterology.* 1998;115(1):42-49.

WHAT ARE THE CHOICES FOR THERAPEUTIC TRIALS (DOSES AND LENGTH OF TRIAL) IN PATIENTS WITH REFLUX SYMPTOMS? DOES THIS MEAN THAT YOU STOP PPIS IF THEY ARE NOT EFFECTIVE?

The choices for therapeutic trials are myriad, debated, and unfortunately not systematically studied to my satisfaction. As true diagnostic _tests_, therapeutic trials have fallen short of their expected promise and whereas easy and expedient compared to diagnostic testing have limits and should not be indefinite as often is the case in practice. I have found several clinical observations to be helpful in planning therapeutic trials. Immediate relief of symptoms (day 1, 2, or 3) is extremely unusual when encountering a new patient. Changing proton pump inhibitors is rarely effective on an empiric basis. Increasing the dose is likely useful only if the initial response is clearly positive. I follow these principles.

If the patient presents with heartburn and/or regurgitation (typical symptoms), I would support a 2- to 4-week trial of once-daily dose of proton pump inhibitor, usually given in the morning before breakfast. As best I can interpret available data, symptom response increases for at least 2 weeks, and in most has reached somewhat of a plateau after 4 weeks. This is in contradistinction to healing, which does not peak until well after 4 weeks. In general, I find that the longer the initial trial, the better understanding I have for what it will take to manage the patient long term. I do not advocate extending the trial beyond 4 weeks, nor do I typically increase the dose empirically in treating typical symptoms unless I have a clear (greater than 50%) progressive improvement. Although switching drugs, changing dose timing to before the evening meal, adding an H_2 blocker all have their support, I consider these part of long-term management or maintenance and not part of a therapeutic trial. So, if I am not happy with the response at 4 weeks, I would do a work up. Whether I stop the PPI depends upon the patient. If my clinical suspicion of GERD is sufficient to treat empirically, I do not eliminate GERD as a diagnosis and stop drug purely based on a therapeutic trial.

Several lines of evidence suggest a different approach to atypical (non-heartburn) presentations. A lower incremental response to once-daily therapy has been observed for all extraesophageal symptoms and many feel are the most difficult. It is in this group that I use the longest "trial," 8 to 12 weeks of twice-daily proton pump inhibitor. This is the best compromise for most patients in my clinical experience. A more rapid response is gratifying and absolutely no improvement after 4 to 8 weeks suggests a low likelihood of GERD in my experience; but again, little harm will come to the patient—either physical or emotional—by waiting and in my experience reduces and focuses diagnostic testing. Again, I do not stop drugs and tell the patient they do not have GERD based purely on empiric trial.

Bibliography

Castell DO, Katz PO. The acid suppression test for unexplained chest pain. *Gastroenterology.* 1998;115(1):222-224.

DeVault KR, Castell DO. American College of Gastroenterology. Updated guidelines for the diagnosis and treatment of gastroesophageal reflux disease. *Am J Gastroenterol.* 2005;100(1):190-200.

Fass R, Fennerty MB, Ofman JJ, et al. The clinical and economic value of a short course of omeprazole in patients with noncardiac chest pain. *Gastroenterology.* 1998;115(1):42-49.

Metz DC, Inadomi JM, Howden CW, et al. On-demand therapy for GERD. *Am J Gastroenterol.* 2007;102(3):642-653.

WHAT IS THE MECHANISM OF ACTION OF ANTISECRETORY THERAPY FOR GERD?

Antisecretory agents (H$_2$ receptor antagonists [H$_2$RAs] and proton pump inhibitors [PPIs]) inhibit gastric acid secretion and raise intragastric pH decreasing the damaging potential of the refluxate. The number of hours the pH is >4.0 is considered an efficacy measure of the inhibition of acid secretion. When intragastric pH <4.0, pepsinogen is activated to pepsin, which can exacerbate esophageal mucosal damage caused by the acid. A prospective study has found that healing of erosive esophagitis symptom relief by acid-suppressive agents is related to the duration of gastric acid suppression over a 24-hour period (Tables 15-1 and 15-2).

Parietal cells located within the mucosa of the stomach are responsible for acid secretion. These cells produce an average of two liters of acidic gastric juice per day. Occupation of the receptors on the basal-lateral membrane of the parietal cell can stimulate acid secretion. Gastrin release is stimulated by food. Acetylcholine is released via stimulation of the vagus nerve by the sight, smell, and taste of food. These two receptors stimulate the enterochromaffin-like (ECL) cells to release histamine. Histamine stimulates the generation of cyclic adenosine 3′,5′-monophosphate (cAMP), which stimulates acid production. Regardless of the primary stimulation, the production of acid through H$^+$,K$^+$-ATPase (the proton pump) is the final common path of acid secretion. It is this step that is inhibited by PPIs.

Optimal use of PPIs is aided by an understanding of their pharmacology. PPIs are weak bases, incompletely absorbed, with short half-lives (0.6 to 1.9 hours). They accumulate and activate in an acid environment at the secretory canalicular surface of the parietal cell. In this environment, the inactive benzimidazole of the PPI is converted to a cationic tetracyclic sulfonamide, which covalently bind to cysteines residues on the alpha subunit of the H$^+$,K$^+$-ATPase enzyme, irreversibly inhibiting acid production of the bound cell in

Table 15-1

Relationship Between Percent Time pH >4.0 and Healing of Erosive Esophagitis Grades C and D

Healing status	Mean % time intragastric pH >4.0
Healed	61.3%
Not healed	42.2%

$P = .002$.
Healing = 69.9% at 4 weeks.
Reprinted from Katz PO, Ginsberg GG, Hoyle PE, Sostek MB, Monyak JT, Silberg DG. Relationship between intragastric acid control and healing status in the treatment of moderate to severe erosive oesophagitis. *Aliment Pharmacol Ther.* 2007;25(5):617-628. With permission from Blackwell Scientific Publications.

Table 15-2

Relationship Between Esophageal Acid Control and Healing Status

Healing status	Mean % time intragastric pH > 4.0
Healed	95.2%
Not healed	88.9%

$P = .006$.
Healing = 69.9% at 4 weeks.
Reprinted from Katz PO, Ginsberg GG, Hoyle PE, Sostek MB, Monyak JT, Silberg DG. Relationship between intragastric acid control and healing status in the treatment of moderate to severe erosive oesophagitis. *Aliment Pharmacol Ther.* 2007;25(5):617-628. With permission from Blackwell Scientific Publications.

about 70% of active pumps. Cysteine binding differences between PPIs may effect pharmacokinetics but offer little difference in clinical effects. Secretory capacity is restored when new pumps (H^+,K^+-ATPase molecules) are converted from their inactive status in the tubulovesicle to their active form at the canalicular surface, which occurs on average in 36 to 72 hours. As a class, PPIs suppress daytime, nocturnal, and meal-stimulated acid secretion. The degree of acid inhibition with PPIs does not correlate with plasma concentration but to the area under the curve (AUC). The slower a PPI is cleared from the plasma, the more of it is available to be delivered to the proton pump. The clinical implications of this are difficult to discern.

Proton pump inhibitors only activate proton pumps. Because no pumps are active at any given time, a single dose of a PPI does not inhibit all pumps and does not result in profound inhibition of acid secretion. Acid secretion by these proton pumps will, therefore, be inhibited with subsequent PPI doses, taking 5 to 7 days to achieve a steady state with a PPI. Acid inhibition is never total because of continual synthesis of new proton pumps. If PPIs are administered twice daily, then more active proton pumps will be exposed to the drug, and steady-state inhibition of gastric acid secretion will be achieved more rapidly and will be more complete.

Bibliography

Katz PO. Medical therapy for GERD in 2007. *Rev in Gastroenterol Disord.* 2007;25(5):617-628.

Katz PO, Ginsberg GG, Hoyle PE, Sostek MB, Monyak JT, Silberg DG. Relationship between intragastric acid control and healing status in the treatment of moderate to severe erosive oesophagitis. *Aliment Pharmacol Ther.* 2007;25(5):617-628.

A Pharmaceutical Rep Tells Me That PPIs Often Fail Because Patients Do Not Take Them As Directed. Is It True That Some PPIs Need To Be Given Before Meals, But Others Do Not?

All available proton pump inhibitors (PPIs) are indicated for once-daily dosing, usually in the morning. Although food has different effects on the bioavailability of each molecule and meal timing may not affect bioavailability of rabeprazole or pantoprazole, it is my practice to recommend that all PPIs be given prior to meals for optimal efficacy. This is based on the concepts outlined in Question 15 and results of an intragastric pH study performed in our laboratory in which significantly superior daytime pH control (time intragastric pH >4) was seen when the PPI was taken before breakfast, compared to an empty stomach in the morning with no food until noon (Figure 16-1).

However, some patients, in particular those with extraesophageal symptoms or complicated disease, need more than a single daily dose of PPI. In these cases, splitting the dose and giving a PPI twice daily, before breakfast and dinner, provides superior intragastric pH control, particularly at night, when compared to a double dose given once daily. Control in daytime pH was similar regardless of when a PPI is given; however, nocturnal pH control is significantly improved with the twice-daily regimen compared to double dose once daily (Figure 16-2).

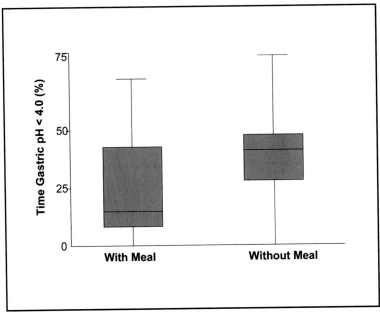

Figure 16-1. Improved intragastric pH control when proton pump inhibitor is given before breakfast and a breakfast meal is ingested. I routinely recommend before meal dosing, regardless of which proton pump inhibitor is chosen as this eliminates any issue of meal timing and is easy for the patient to remember. The drug can be taken when the patient wakes up, while they are preparing a meal, or while waiting for the meal they order in a restaurant.

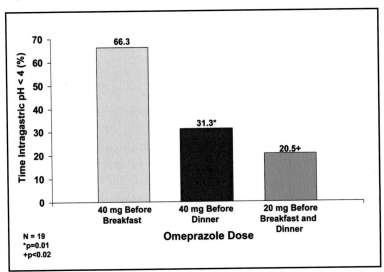

Figure 16-2. Improved nocturnal pH control with a twice-daily dose compared to double dose once daily and improvement in nocturnal control with an evening dose compared to morning, a useful strategy if the patient will comply. (Reprinted from Hatlebakk JG, Katz PO, Kuo B, Castell DO. Nocturnal gastric acidity and acid breakthrough on different regimens of omeprazole 40 mg daily. *Aliment Pharmacol Ther.* 1998;12:1235-1240, with permission from Blackwell Scientific Publications.)

Table 16-1

Percent Time pH > 4 Overnight With Bedtime Dosing of PPIs

Treatment	22:00 to 24:00 hours	First half of the night 22:00 to 02:00 hours	22:00 to 04:00 hours	Entire night time period 22:00 to 06:00 hours
IR-OME 40 mg	32.3 (6.6-94.1)	51.9 (16.8 – 88.7)	62.6 (26.0-88.1)	53.4 (31.3-90.3)
Lansoprazole 30 mg	0.0 (0.0-0.3)+	12.0 (0.0-32.1)+	26.6 (2.8-43.9)+	34.2 (13.3-52.2)+
Esomeprazole 40 mg	0.1 (0.0-14.8)+	30.1 (5.1-48.6)+	46.5 (29.5-64.1)	54.9 (38.2-68.6)

Reprinted from Katz PO, Koch FK, Ballard ED, et al. Comparison of the effects of immediate-release omeprazole oral suspension, delayed-release lansoprazole capsules and delayed-release esomeprazole capsules on nocturnal gastric acidity after bedtime dosing in patients with night-time GERD symptoms. *Aliment Pharmacol Ther.* 2007;25:197-205.

All 5 available agents are extremely effective and safe and are each reasonable choices for initial therapy. In fact, the choice of initial therapy often depends on cost considerations in addition to efficacy. Each makes claim to subtle differences in speed of onset of symptom control, bioavailability, and drug interactions, though few direct head-to-head comparisons of these subtle differences are published. Therefore, beginning therapy with a single daily dose given before breakfast is preferred. The majority of patients will respond to once-daily dosing, achieving effective healing of erosive esophagitis and symptom relief, regardless of the PPI chosen for initial therapy. If treatment is not as successful as desired, patients should be carefully queried about dose timing, particularly the relationship to meals. Patients are too often taking PPIs in the morning and not eating breakfast or taking their drug before bed on an empty stomach. A small adjustment in timing, or simply eating breakfast, may improve outcome. In patients with nighttime symptoms, an evening dose before dinner may be effective. Delayed-release PPIs should not be given before bed on an empty stomach as they do not effectively control intragastric pH in the early part of the sleeping period when the majority of nighttime reflux occurs (see Questions 9 and 10). An evening dose of a delayed-release PPI should control intragastric pH into the critical part of the sleeping period and be sufficient for most patients. Patients in whom a bedtime dose of a PPI is desired, the newest PPI, immediate-release omeprazole sodium bicarbonate (IR-OME; Zegerid) may be considered. Available in capsule and powder form, the 40-mg dose given at bedtime has been shown to be superior to pantoprazole 40 mg given at dinner in control of overnight pH. In a recent study, comparing IR-OME 40 mg suspension, lansoprazole 30 mg, esomeprazole 40 mg given at 10:00 pm on an empty stomach (last meal at 5:00 pm) for 7 days found that IR-OME was superior to the others in speed of overnight pH control and sustained pH control in the first 4 hours of the sleeping period compared to both lansoprazole and esomeprazole (Table 16-1). Sustained daytime control may not be sufficient with IR-OME as a single dose at night. If a higher dose is really needed, the patient should be treated with twice daily PPI, before breakfast and dinner. Immediate-release omeprazole at bedtime may be used in lieu of the evening dose a delayed-release PPI if nocturnal symptoms are not adequately relieved.

Bibliography

Hatlebakk JG, Katz PO, Camacho-Lobato L, Castell DO. Proton pump inhibitors: better acid suppression when taken before a meal than without a meal. *Aliment Pharmacol Ther.* 2000;14(10):1267-1272.

Hatlebakk JG, Katz PO, Kuo B, Castell DO. Nocturnal gastric acidity and acid breakthrough on different regimens of omeprazole 40 mg daily. *Aliment Pharmacol Ther.* 1998;12:1235-1240.

17

WHAT ARE THE SO-CALLED EXTRAESOPHAGEAL MANIFESTATIONS OF GERD?

Alhough heartburn and regurgitation are the most common and typical symptoms of gastroesophageal reflux disease (GERD), several laryngeal, pharyngeal, and pulmonary symptoms have also been associated with this very prevalent disease. The laryngeal symptoms include chronic cough, hoarseness, throat clearing, globus, and numerous others. The symptoms, lumped into the category laryngopharyngeal reflux (LPR), can result in tissue injury manifest as posterior laryngitis, vocal cord nodules, laryngeal edema, granulomas, contact ulcers, sinusitis, and even dental caries. Small reports have demonstrated an association of LPR with laryngeal carcinoma, laryngospasm, and laryngeal stenosis. GERD has also been associated with multiple pulmonary symptoms, the most common of which is bronchial asthma. The very complex disease, idiopathic pulmonary fibrosis (IPF), has been linked to GERD as has recurrent aspiration pneumonia chronic bronchitis and bronchiectasis.

The pathogenesis of these extraesophageal symptoms is multifactorial, revolving around 2 major mechanisms—a vagovagal reflex and microaspiration of gastric contents. Ultimately, the indictment of GERD as the etiologic factor for these symptoms and signs is difficult as neither endoscopy nor prolonged reflux monitoring have shown consistent evidence of either esophageal injury or abnormal reflux frequency (distal, proximal, hypopharyngeal, or any combination). Controlled trials of antireflux therapy are few and the available results conflicting. Nevertheless, gastroenterologists and other specialists are often confronted with difficult to manage patients with these so-called extraesophageal symptoms considered to be due to GERD.

Two principal hypotheses have been suggested for the pathogenesis of this condition, aspiration of gastric contents resulting in direct contact with the upper airway and a vagovagal reflex.

Extraesophageal symptoms of GERD are common in patients with GERD. This has been documented in an excellent population-based study. An increase in many of the so-called signs and symptoms of extraesophageal disease were seen in patients with both frequent and infrequent GERD compared to those without GERD. At least one atypical symptom was present in almost 80% of individuals with frequent (at least weekly) GERD symptoms compared to only 48% of those without typical GERD symptoms. Using logistic regression, typical GERD symptoms were associated with noncardiac chest pain, dysphagia, globus, and dyspepsia. A study using a large Veteran's Administration database found an increased odds ratio of sinusitis, pharyngitis, aphonia, laryngitis, laryngeal stenosis, and asthma in patients with reflux esophagitis compared to matched controls. An increased frequency of IPF and other pulmonary symptoms was noted as well. The strongest associations were with asthma and IPF. In this study, approximately 17% of patients with esophagitis had an extraesophageal manifestation of GERD. GERD has been diagnosed in as many as 75% of patients with chronic hoarseness and laryngeal stenosis. It has been seen in 70% to 80% of patients with asthma and up to 20% with chronic cough. These collective studies suggest a variable but clear increase in extraesophageal symptoms in patients with GERD. Of particular note, is that patients with extraesophageal manifestations of GERD appear to have a lower frequency of heartburn than would be expected, with many patients presenting with little or no heartburn even when aggressively sought in history taking.

Bibliography

Irwin RS, Curley FJ, French CL. Chronic cough. The spectrum and frequency of causes, key components, of the diagnostic evaluation, and outcome of specific therapy. *Am Rev Respir Dis.* 1990;141:640-647.

Locke R III, Talley N, Fett S, et al. Prevalence and clinical spectrum of gastroesophageal reflux: a population based study in Olmstead County, Minnesota. *Gastroenterology.* 1997;112:1448-1456.

Vaezi MF. Laryngitis and gastroesophageal reflux disease: increasing prevalence or poor diagnostic tests? *Am J Gastroenterol.* 2004;99:786-788.

IS THE DIAGNOSTIC APPROACH TO GERD PATIENTS DIFFERENT THAN PATIENTS WITH TYPICAL SYMPTOMS OF HEARTBURN AND REGURGITATION?

Although the relationship between GERD and the above mentioned pulmonary and laryngeal symptoms has been well documented, the diagnosis of GERD remains difficult in the individual patient. Specifically, many of the signs and symptoms of laryngopharyngeal reflux (LPR) overlap with other diseases and may be seen in normal controls. Asthma, chronic cough, and idiopathic pulmonary fibrosis (IPF) are common clinical entities as is GERD in the general population. Therefore, a multipronged approach including a thorough history, therapeutic trial of antisecretory therapy, endoscopy, and prolonged reflux monitoring need to be used together to arrive at an adequate diagnosis.

Pulmonary symptoms suggesting GERD include nighttime cough, and/or increase in asthma symptoms after meals, or recumbent. Adult onset asthma, nonallergic asthma, and nonresponsive asthma should heighten suspicion of GERD. In rare cases, a reflux episode (heartburn) will herald an asthma attack. Endoscopy is abnormal in less than 40%. Barium studies are nonspecific, though a large hiatal hernia with reflux into the proximal esophagus should arouse suspicion. Esophageal pH monitoring is the most effective test to document the presence of abnormal esophageal acid exposure, proximal and/or hypopharyngeal exposure, and associate symptoms with reflux. Unfortunately, studies show variable results with the former and it is extremely rare that reflux will produce a single episode of wheezing.

There are few direct clues to the presence of GERD in patients with suspected IPF, chronic bronchitis, or recurrent aspiration pneumonia, therefore an aggressive search for reflux should be undertaken in patients who have these problems as proton pump inhibitors may make management easier. Patients with chronic cough should have a chest x-ray, a good history for documentation of angiotensin-converting enzyme (ACE) inhibitor use and smoking and likely will need multispecialty exams to rule out sinusitis, postnasal drip, and asthma. Although GERD has been documented to be the third most common cause of chronic cough in nonsmokers, the aforementioned problems often overlap and may need to be treated in concert. In fact, more than one cause is usually found for refractory asthma, though GERD may be the most common cause.

The symptoms most commonly associated with LPR have multiple etiologies. The most common laryngeal abnormalities seen in GERD include erythema and edema of the vocal cords as well as the posterior glottis. Vocal cord granulomas and other laryngeal findings including erythema of the posterior vocal cords, contact ulcers, vocal cord polyps, and subglottic stenosis in patients who have been previously intubated have been reported to be associated with GERD. An intriguing study of asymptomatic so-called normal controls found many of these abnormalities to be present, specifically edema and vocal cord erythema. Therefore, it is difficult to make a conclusive diagnosis of LPR based entirely on the ENT examination.

An intriguing association between reflux and chronic gingivitis and dental erosions has been documented. A loss of tooth structure, measured by the tooth wear index found that adults diagnosed with GERD had higher tooth wear index scores compared to controls, suggesting that the erosions or tooth decay may be exacerbated by GERD. The progression of these lesions is believed to be slow suggesting that the dentist might query the patient with these problems for the presence of reflux.

The most common approach to the typical GERD patient is to perform endoscopy to evaluate for erosive esophagitis and/or Barrett's esophagus. This approach is not recommended in patients with extraesophageal symptoms as endoscopy is usually normal in these patients. Even if erosive esophagitis is seen it does not prove that the symptoms are due to GERD. Therefore endoscopy should not be routinely performed as it increases cost without major benefit. Endoscopy can be used to screen for Barrett's esophagus in the appropriate patient.

When a gastroenterologist is referred a patient with suspected extraesophageal GERD, they have invariably been on high-dose antisecretory therapy. Thus prolonged reflux monitoring, either with combined multichannel intraluminal impedance/pH or wireless esophageal acid monitoring (Bravo) is the most appropriate diagnostic intervention to consider at this critical juncture. Although prolonged monitoring performed while on antisecretory therapy will most often demonstrate normal esophageal acid control if the patient is on twice-daily prton pump inhibitor (PPI), a well-defined percentage (2% to 10%) will have continued acid reflux with a positive symptom association, and many will demonstrate so called non-acid reflux with a positive symptom association. The presence of proximal or hypopharyngeal reflux is not in and of itself a big diagnostic help though I find it helpful in some situations. Intragastric pH monitoring is not required on a routine basis but may add information in difficult cases.

Therefore it is usually my preference to perform on therapy monitoring with combined intraluminal impedance/pH monitoring to immediately look for both acid and non-acid reflux. If this technology is unavailable, on-therapy esophageal monitoring should be performed, with either Bravo or traditional catheter based electrodes. If the clinical situation dictates, I will stop antisecretory therapy for 7 to 10 days and perform a Bravo study off therapy. I do this in patients sent for surgical evaluation, those in whom I doubt the presence of GERD, any who will not tolerate a catheter and/or when "proof" of the presence or absence of GERD at baseline is needed either for the patient or referring physician. The period off therapy is a good opportunity for the patient to evaluate how much the antisecretory therapy actually helps their symptoms.

Overall, I believe the most efficient and likely beneficial approach to the patient in whom GERD is suspected is a careful therapeutic trial of antisecretory therapy (see Bibliography), with symptom improvement the basis for the correct diagnosis.

Bibliography

Irwin RS, Curley FJ, French CL. Chronic cough. The spectrum and frequency of causes, key components, of the diagnostic evaluation, and outcome of specific therapy. *Am Rev Respir Dis*. 1990;141:640-647.

Locke R III, Talley N, Fett S, et al. Prevalence and clinical spectrum of gastroesophageal reflux: a population based study in Olmstead County, Minnesota. *Gastroenterology*. 1997;112:1448-1456.

Vaezi MF. Laryngitis and gastroesophageal reflux disease: increasing prevalence or poor diagnostic tests? *Am J Gastroenterol*. 2004;99:786-788.

ARE THE THERAPEUTIC CHOICES DIFFERENT FOR THESE PATIENTS AND, IF SO, HOW?

Treatment is based on extending the principles advocated for treating patients with heartburn and erosive esophagitis, observations from available clinical trials and clinical experience.

The most efficient way to determine if symptoms/signs are due to laryngopharyngeal reflux (LPR) or pulmonary-related GERD is to attempt to eliminate the symptom(s) with a high-dose proton pump inhibitor (PPI) trial after other nonreflux causes of these symptoms have been excluded. This is because the weight of the available evidence supports the lack of sufficient sensitivity and specificity of endoscopy and prolonged pH monitoring performed off therapy to make a diagnosis. The former is based on clinical experience and collected series finding well under 30% of patients having an abnormal endoscopy. The latter is highlighted by 2 well-done studies. A large randomized multicenter placebo controlled trial comparing esomeprazole 40 mg twice daily in patients with laryngeal signs and symptoms suspected to be GERD related revealed no predictive value of either distal, proximal, or hypopharyngeal pH monitoring in predicting PPI response. A similar study comparing lansoprazole to placebo in patients with abnormal 24-hour pH and abnormal ENT exam also found little or no positive or negative predictive value of an abnormal pH study in determining clinical response. Although the optimal dose and duration of antisecretory therapy has not been determined, available data evaluating the ability to control intragastric and intraesophageal pH, uncontrolled studies, and clinical observation suggest that an 8- to 16-week trial of PPI twice daily before breakfast and dinner is the most efficient initial step. Some patients will respond relatively quickly so I do my first follow up at 4 weeks. This is particularly evident in patients with chronic cough, as shown in a small study of 17 patients with abnormal distal esophageal acid exposure. Though only 6 (35%) responded, these patients reported striking resolution in

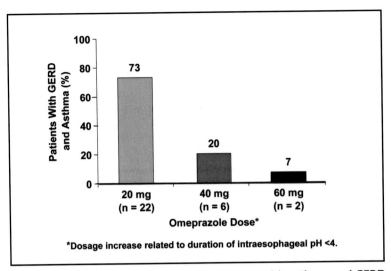

Figure 19-1. Thirty nonsmoking adult patients with asthma and GERD were recruited from the outpatient clinics of a university hospital. Omeprazole dose was titrated until acid suppression was documented normal by 24-hour pH testing. Treatment lasted up to 3 months. A proportion of patients required more than 1 dose of omeprazole to normalize esophageal pH. This provides foundation for high-dose therapy. (Reprinted from Harding SM, Richter JE, Guzzo MR, Schan CA, Alexander RW, Bradley LA. Asthma and gastroesophageal reflux: acid suppressive therapy improved asthma outcome. *Am J Med.* 1996;100:395-405, with permission from Excerpta Medica.)

their symptoms within 2 weeks of omeprazole (40 mg bid) therapy, which was sustained over 1 year. This approach, if successful, avoids the cost of diagnostic procedures and limits them to those who don't respond. Incomplete responders may need still longer treatment, so unless there is absolutely no response, I would continue the initial treatment for 12 weeks. Treatment response may be slow and illustrate the need for high-dose therapy (Figures 19-1 and 19-2).

If symptoms are relieved, a maintenance program can be developed. Relapse is frequent when therapy is stopped and with no long-term data available, I continue the twice-daily dose of PPI for a minimum of 6 months. It is my experience that step-down therapy is rarely successful so I do not encourage this approach. Antireflux surgery is a long-term option to consider, especially in those with clear aspiration symptoms, perhaps the refractory asthmatic, and should be considered prior to lung transplant if the patient has GERD. Surgery has decreased efficacy in relief of extraesophageal GERD symptoms compared to the results with heartburn and regurgitation. Though not compared head to head, in my opinion offer similar outcome to long-term medical therapy in most cases of extraesophageal disease. Endoscopic therapy has not been studied in extraesophageal disease so I do not recommend it. In the final analysis, the average patient stays on long-term therapy with high-dose PPI if they respond.

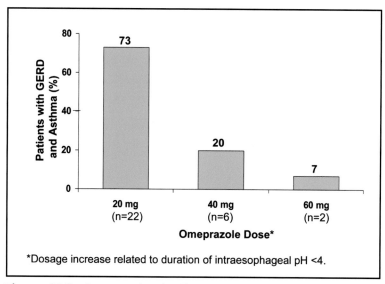

*Dosage increase related to duration of intraesophageal pH <4.

Figure 19-2. Omeprazole significantly reduced asthma symptom scores in responders over a 3-month period. Not all patients will respond even if they have documented abnormal pH monitoring study. (Reprinted from Harding SM, Richter JE, Guzzo MR, Schan CA, Alexander RW, Bradley LA. Asthma and gastroesophageal reflux: acid suppressive therapy improved asthma outcome. *Am J Med.* 1996;100:395-405, with permission from Excerpta Medica.)

Conclusions

The association of head and neck, pulmonary symptoms, and gastroesophageal reflux disease is real, but the patients are difficult. A rigorous, comprehensive approach to the patient is required, accepting that many will have more than 1 etiology, including GERD, for their symptoms. Aggressive antisecretory therapy, with careful evaluation with prolonged reflux monitoring both on and off therapy, is often required to adequately evaluate the patient. A satisfying outcome is often achieved when this careful approach is practiced.

Bibliography

Irwin RS, Curley FJ, French CL. Chronic cough. The spectrum and frequency of causes, key components, of the diagnostic evaluation, and outcome of specific therapy. *Am Rev Respir Dis.* 1990;141:640-647.

Locke R III, Talley N, Fett S, et al. Prevalence and clinical spectrum of gastroesophageal reflux: a population based study in Olmstead County, Minnesota. *Gastroenterology.* 1997;112:1448-1456.

Vaezi MF. Laryngitis and gastroesophageal reflux disease: increasing prevalence or poor diagnostic tests? *Am J Gastroenterol.* 2004;99:786-788.

A Patient With Long-Standing GERD Is Asymptomatic on a Once-Daily PPI. He Wants to Know if He Needs to Take His Medication "for the Rest of His Life." Address the Long-term Maintenance Therapy for GERD.

You are faced with a patient who has had an excellent response to once-a-day proton pump inhibitor with complete relief of reflux symptoms. In answering the question, "Does he need to take medication for the rest of his life?" it is important to put into perspective the natural history of gastroesophageal reflux disease, both from the standpoint of symptomatic recurrence, recurrence of erosive disease, and the potential for complications long term (Figure 20-1). It is very clear that this person, regardless of his age, gender, or ethnic background, will have some recurrence of symptoms if therapy is completely stopped. This is illustrated quite well in multiple trials. If one looks carefully at a cohort of patients who are treated systematically with a proton pump inhibitor up to the equivalent of omeprazole 20 mg once daily and are rendered asymptomatic and followed for 6 months for the presence of recurrent symptoms, a symptomatic relapse will occur in over 80% of patients. This is independent of the presence or absence of erosive esophagitis at baseline. If one looks carefully at these patient cohorts, symptomatic relapse is somewhat more likely if at the time of original diagnosis the patient had erosive disease. In my experience, however, this is not clinically important. In reality, I would tell this patient that his symptoms would recur and that it was highly likely that he would want some

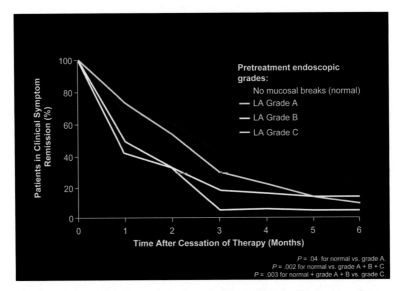

Figure 20-1. GERD is a chronic condition that is likely to relapse. When therapy is stopped, symptoms will relapse. Few, if any, will not require some long-term intervention. (Reprinted from Lundell L, Dent J, Bennett JR, et al. Endoscopic assessment of oesophagitis: clinical and functional correlates and further validation of the Los Angeles classification. *Gut.* 1999;45:172-180, with permission from the British Medical Association.)

form of therapy (continuous or on demand) to decrease, relieve, or eliminate symptoms. If one looks strictly at the likelihood of complications, it is very unlikely that after an initial diagnosis is made and symptoms are relieved that serious complication will develop long term. Though there is some variation, in reality there is little evidence to show that nonerosive reflux disease will progress even if symptoms are allowed to recur and are treated on an as-needed basis. Although it is also clear that patients with severe erosive esophagitis (grades C and D) and potentially any grade of erosive esophagitis is likely to recur, the progression to peptic stricture, Barrett's esophagus, or the more serious complication of adenocarcinoma would be unusual if Barrett's esophagus was eliminated from diagnostic consideration. In reality, patients with erosive esophagitis, grades C and D, will "do better" with continuous therapy; however, there are many who do not require this type of intervention.

Thus, I would counsel the patient that symptoms are likely to recur, make an assessment of the risk profile for the development of Barrett's esophagus, and recommend screening in light of that risk and discuss with the patient the long-term options relative to medical therapy. If there were a concern about the cost, side effects, and/or inconvenience of long-term medical therapy, this is a reasonable time to discuss the pros and cons of antireflux surgery. In this light, the discussion would center around both the initial success of surgery, the potential for relapse over time (approximately 20% to 30% at 7 years), and the potential side effects of same. I would have the discussion relative to risk of complications, emphasizing that there was no clear evidence that continued therapy and/or antireflux surgery would prevent those. With this information, a patient can make an informed decision about the desire for maintenance therapy and what type they would prefer.

There are 3 options available for long-term medical management of patients with gastroesophageal reflux disease, keeping in mind that the goals of therapy are relief and/or resolution of symptoms, optimizing health-related quality of life, and, as mentioned above, prevention of complications. The 3 available options for patients are continuous long-term therapy, true on-demand intermittent therapy, and so-called "threshold" therapy. In reality, those patients on so-called continuous medical therapy do not take their medications on a regular basis and, as such, are on their own form of on-demand or intermittent therapy. Although distinguishing between these types of therapy may seem semantic, they in reality are different. In on-demand therapy, the patient will wait for symptoms to return, taking some form of medication only for as long as symptoms are present. In intermittent therapy, the patient will take short courses of medical treatment for a defined period of time (days, weeks, or months) and then stops. Threshold therapy—the patient titrates their medication to the lowest frequency to control symptoms (every other, every third, every fourth, or other form of regular therapy)—has not been systematically studied. Ultimately the average patient simply takes their medication on their own schedule.

Multiple-outcome measures have been used to evaluate on-demand and intermittent therapy and understanding these end points enhances our understanding of what our patients might experience. One can use the number of heartburn-free days, the number of rescue antacids taken, cost, relapse of esophagitis, or willingness to continue or discontinue the type of therapy randomized to. Thus, it is impossible to absolutely know which patient will do well with on-demand or other form of noncontinuous therapy until it is tried.

Bibliography

Lundell L, Dent J, Bennett JR, et al. Endoscopic assessment of oesophagitis: clinical and functional correlates and further validation of the Los Angeles classification. *Gut.* 1999;45:172-180.

Norman Hansen A, Bergheim R, Fagertun H, et al. A randomized prospective study comparing the effectiveness of esomeprazole treatment strategies in clinical practice for 6 months in the management of patients with symptoms of gastroesophageal reflux disease. *Int J Clin Pract.* 2005;59(6):665-671.

Sjostedt S, Befrits R, Sylvan A, et al. Daily treatment with esomeprazole is superior to that taken on-demand for maintenance of healed erosvie esophagitis. *Aliment Pharmacol Ther.* 2005;22:183-191.

WHAT IS THE ROLE OF AN ON-DEMAND TREATMENT IN MAINTENANCE? WHO IS THE BEST CANDIDATE?

There are 3 options available for long-term medical management of patients with gastroesophageal reflux disease, keeping in mind that the goals of therapy are relief and/or resolution of symptoms, optimizing health-related quality of life and, as mentioned above, prevention of complications. The 3 available options for patients are continuous long-term therapy, true on-demand intermittent therapy, and so-called "threshold" therapy (Figure 21-1). In reality, those patients on so-called continuous medical therapy do not take their medications on a regular basis and, as such, are on their own form of on-demand or intermittent therapy. Although distinguishing between these types of therapy may seem semantic, they in reality are different. In on-demand therapy, the patient will wait for symptoms to return, taking some form of medication only for as long as symptoms are present. In intermittent therapy, the patient will take short courses of medical treatment for a defined period of time (days, weeks, or months) and then stops. Threshold therapy—the patient titrates their medication to the lowest frequency to control symptoms (every other, every third, every fourth, or other form of regular therapy)—has not been systematically studied. Ultimately the average patient simply takes their medication on their own schedule.

Multiple-outcome measures have been used to evaluate on-demand and intermittent therapy and understanding these end points enhances our understanding of what our patients might experience. One can use the number of heartburn-free days, the number of rescue antacids taken, cost, relapse of esophagitis, or willingness to continue or discontinue the type of therapy randomized to. Thus, it is impossible to absolutely know which patient will do well with on-demand or other form of noncontinuous therapy until it is tried.

It is useful to know that patients who complain of mild heartburn more than once or twice per week have a diminution in quality of life. It is also clear that for many patients, symptom episodes are relatively short and that the "episodes" can be shortened by

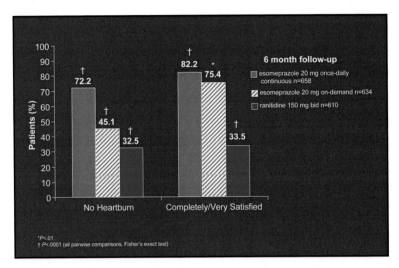

Figure 21-1. Once-daily continuous versus on-demand therapy: heartburn and patient satisfaction. Study shows that continuous acid suppression offers best overall outcome. Ultimately, daily treatment or not becomes a patient choice. (Reprinted from Norman Hansen A, Bergheim R, Fagertun H, et al. A randomized prospective study comparing the effectiveness of esomeprazole treatment strategies in clinical practice for 6 months in the management of patients with symptoms of gastroesophageal reflux disease. *Int J Clin Pract.* 2005;59[6]:665-671, with permission from Blackwell Publishing.)

rapidly initiating treatment. It is also clear that patients wish to be in control of their own therapy and often titrate their treatment to symptom prevalence and severity. As such, patients on long-term proton pump inhibitor (PPI) therapy often take their treatment less than 50% of the study days even if they have erosive esophagitis.

In reality, patients will continue on-demand therapy despite periodic symptom recurrence in most studies in which this outcome measure is assessed. Although there are no consensus recommendations, it is my opinion that patients with nonerosive reflux disease can easily be put into an on-demand maintenance program without concern of complications. This is likely the case in patients with mild erosive esophagitis (grades A and B) as well. Although this is in many ways controversial as the erosive disease is more likely to relapse with on-demand than so-called continuous therapy, symptomatic relapse rates and patient satisfaction do not differ dramatically in those that recur and those that do not. I would not recommend on-demand therapy in patients with severe esophagitis (Los Angeles grades C and D), those with Barrett's esophagus, extraesophageal manifestations of GERD, or patients with a history of peptic stricture. Though arguably one might say that I do not have the data to show that these patients need continuous therapy to prevent complications, it is my strong clinical impression that symptom relapse and decrement in quality of life are less and substantially so when these latter groups take continuous therapy.

Finally, how might one approach the patient who is empirically treated, has successful symptom remission, and wants to know whether he or she needs to continue with daily therapy? I would say that a screening endoscopy to rule out Barrett's should be performed and if Barrett's is not present, then on-demand therapy would be reasonable, with continuous therapy always possible if relapses were frequent (Figures 21-2 and 21-3).

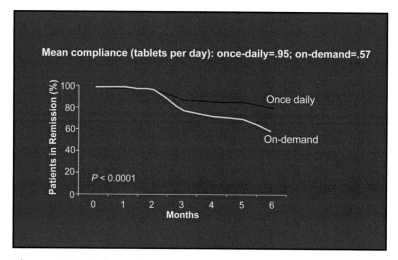

Figure 21-2. Endoscopic remission at 6 months. Relapse is more likely if on-demand treatment is used; however, many will do quite well. (Reprinted from Sjöstedt S, Befrits R, Sylvan A, et al. Daily treatment with esomeprazole is superior to that taken on-demand for maintenance of healed erosive esophagitis. *Aliment Pharmacol Ther.* 2005;22:183-191, with permission from Blackwell Scientific Publications.)

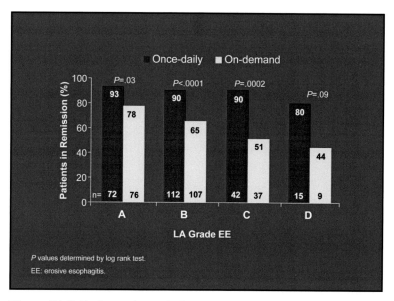

Figure 21-3. Endoscopic remission at 6 months: effects of baseline severity. Study suggests that those with more severe disease at baseline may be better served with daily therapy. Unfortunately, few did early endoscopy and symptoms were not evaluated. (Reprinted from Sjöstedt S, Befrits R, Sylvan A, et al. Daily treatment with esomeprazole is superior to that taken on-demand for maintenance of healed erosive esophagitis. *Aliment Pharmacol Ther.* 2005;22:183-191, with permission from Blackwell Scientific Publications.)

Ultimately, the choice in many ways should be left to the patient and the decision for type of maintenance therapy should be based on patient preference, symptoms, quality of life, and cost.

Bibliography

Lundell L, Dent J, Bennett JR, et al. Endoscopic assessment of oesophagitis: clinical and functional correlates and further validation of the Los Angeles classification. *Gut.* 1999;45:172-180.

Norman Hansen A, Bergheim R, Fagertun H, et al. A randomized prospective study comparing the effectiveness of esomeprazole treatment strategies in clinical practice for 6 months in the management of patients with symptoms of gastroesophageal reflux disease. *Int J Clin Pract.* 2005;59(6):665-671.

Sjöstedt S, Befrits R, Sylvan A, et al. Daily treatment with esomeprazole is superior to that taken on-demand for maintenance of healed erosvie esophagitis. *Aliment Pharmacol Ther.* 2005;22:183-191.

WHAT IS THE ROLE OF PROKINETIC AGENTS IN THE TREATMENT OF GERD, AND HOW DO I KNOW WHICH ONE TO USE?

Conceptually, a "promotility or motility-altering agent" is still held up as the ideal agent to treat GERD. Addressing the underlying pathophysiologic defects of the lower esophageal sphincter, augmenting esophageal clearance, and increasing gastric emptying would indeed constitute the ideal therapy. Unfortunately the effects of prokinetic agents on lower esophageal sphincter pressure and esophageal clearance are transient at best, and accelerating gastric emptying has not been documented in any study I am aware of to improve symptoms in GERD patients. Since the withdrawal of cisapride, metoclopramide remains the only approved agent available and it has limited therapeutic efficacy and an unfavorable side effect profile.

Clinical trials have found equivalent efficacy of metoclopramide compared to H_2 receptor antagonists (H_2RAs) in relieving heartburn and other GERD symptoms. At a dose of 10 mg 4 times daily, it is more effective than placebo in improving symptoms; however, it is not very effective in healing of erosive esophagitis. Combination prokinetic and H_2RA has shown benefit over either alone but pales in contrast to even once-a-day proton pump inhibitor (PPI). Anxiety, agitation, confusion, motor restlessness, hallucinations, and drowsiness are the most common side effects, seen in up to 20% to 30% of patients. Depression and tardive dyskinesia (potentially irreversible) are the most serious side effects. Side effects appear to be dose related and higher in the elderly. Maintenance studies have suggested a small improvement in outcomes when cisapride was added to omeprazole once daily compared to omeprazole alone; however, this has not been demonstrated with metoclopramide and is not as effective as twice-daily proton pump inhibitors. Though still often used empirically in combination with PPI twice daily in difficult to manage patients, I rarely see efficacy in this setting and do not do this in my practice. If there were a use for this agent in GERD, it would be in those with documented gastroparesis, especially patients with scleroderma, the only place I use it in my practice. Even then, antisecretory therapy is usually sufficient if used in high doses as needed. Clinicians should be careful when prescribing this drug long term. Careful monitoring for side effects must be documented to avoid litigation.

Domperidone, a dopamine agonist that does not cross the blood-brain barrier, has few of the central dopaminergic side effects of metoclopramide. It is available outside the United States and still is used by patients who can obtain it. It should not be administered with antisecretory agents or antacids because reduced gastric acidity may impair its absorption. Efficacy studies suggest similarity to H_2RAs (ranitidine and famotidine) in symptom relief and in promotion of esophageal healing. Hyperprolactinemia, nipple tenderness, galactorrhea, and amenorrhea are the most common side effects of this agent, which in my opinion rarely helps patients with GERD. I do not use it at all in my practice though will not tell patients to stop it if they have obtained it elsewhere.

Tegaserod, a selective partial 5HT4 (5-hydroxytryptamine[4]) agonist, was approved for irritable bowel syndrome and constipation. An early study suggested efficacy in reducing reflux; however, no substantial clinical trials have been produced to date to support its use. In my experience, it was occasionally useful in patients with functional heartburn but not GERD. The drug is currently not marketed in the United States. Erythromycin, a motilin agonist that can improve gastric emptying, is not useful in reflux. Bethanecol, a cholinergic agent, also has a limited role, and is rarely used in adult practice. Overall, prokinetic agents have fallen well short of expectations and play little role in the management of the GERD patient today. As noted above, I rarely use them.

A drug class that offers promise are those in the class of γ-aminobutyric acid (GABA) agonists. The available agent, baclofen, used in treatment of some neurologic diseases, has been shown to reduce the number of transient lower esophageal sphincter relaxations in the postprandial period and to reduce reflux. I have had some success with this drug in treating regurgitation in patients with non-acid reflux documented by impedance. I start with a low dose of 5 mg once to 3 times daily and increasing to 10 mg 3 times daily. The drug is limited by side effects (nausea, dizziness, drowsiness, etc.) and most cannot tolerate it long term. GABA agonists that do not cross the blood-brain barrier (reducing side effects) are very early in development.

Bibliography

Bright-Asare P, El-Bassoussi M. Cimetidine, metoclopramide or placebo in the treatment of symptomatic gastro-esophageal reflux. *J Clin Gastroenterol*. 1980;2:149.

McCallum RW, Ippoliti AF, Cooner C, et al. A controlled trial of metoclopramide in symptomatic gastroesophageal reflux. *N Engl J Med*. 1977;296:354.

A PATIENT WITH CLASSIC GERD SYMPTOMS IS UNHAPPY WITH HIS CURRENT TREATMENT. WHAT IS THE APPROACH TO A PATIENT WITH CONTINUED SYMPTOMS ON ONCE-DAILY PPI? ON TWICE-DAILY PPI?

A 65-year-old gentleman with classic GERD (heartburn and regurgitation) presents with incomplete symptom relief on once-daily proton pump inhibitors (PPIs). He has endoscopic findings of erosive esophagitis and Barrett's (biopsy confirmed). Once-daily PPI improves his symptoms by about 65%, and whereas an increase in PPI dose results in complete daytime symptom relief, some residual nighttime symptoms remain. The approach to the patient at this point is not straightforward.

We have come to "expect" that the vast majority of patients who present with heart-burn will have effective symptom relief on once-daily PPIs. Although this is true in the vast majority of patients, a clinically important number will fail to have complete symptom relief even after 8 weeks of therapy. A meta-analysis published in 1997 found that PPIs given once daily resulted in 77.4% (±10.4%) of patients with erosive esophagitis being heartburn free after 8 weeks of therapy. In a study specifically evaluating daytime and nighttime heartburn separately after 8 weeks of therapy, patients on omeprazole 20 mg per day reported experiencing heartburn on 11.8% of days and 8% of nights, compared to patients on 30 mg of lansoprazole a day experiencing heartburn 8.6% of days and 6.5% of the nights. Using variations in efficacy measures from relief to complete relief to complete resolution, somewhere between 60% and 85% of patients with erosive esophagitis at baseline reach the measured end point at between 4 and 8 weeks. In the more heterogeneous group of patients with nonerosive reflux (heartburn with a normal endoscopy), complete absence of heartburn is reported in lower frequency (46% to 57%). In this patient population, another efficacy measure is the number of heartburn-free days, which in a single study using esomeprazole was approximately 66% of the days. The latter patients may be a better representation of the universe of patients who receive empiric therapy. Regardless of efficacy measure or initial endoscopic appearance, these results suggest that a core of patients will have incomplete relief even of classic GERD symptoms.

Few would argue that in this setting of a classic presentation of GERD and partial symptom relief on once-daily PPI that increasing his proton pump inhibitor is a straightforward choice. Another consideration would include changing the timing of the once-daily dose to before dinner, based on intragastric pH data showing that overnight intragastric pH control is greater when once-daily PPI is given before the evening meal, compared to the morning. In my experience, this works only when nighttime symptoms are predominant. There are no outcome studies that have tested this option. A bedtime dose of PPI would not be logical with a delayed-release PPI. Omeprazole immediate release (IR) (nonenteric coated granules protected by sodium bicarbonate) has made this choice more logical. This drug provides rapid control of intragastric pH early in the sleeping period with what appears to be sustained control throughout the night at steady state. Overall, it is not clear if sufficient daytime control of pH will be provided with this formulation compared to delayed-release PPIs given before dinner when they would be most effective in overnight pH control. Nevertheless a bedtime dose of omeprazole IR has inherent logic behind it.

What is not clear is whether there is any overall gain from switching to another delayed-release PPI. There is interindividual variability in pH control between PPIs, which provides foundation for a switch (Table 23-1). If a switch in delayed-release PPI is entertained, esomeprazole would be the logical second choice, as intragastric pH control with this agent is usually superior to the others given once daily in the morning (see Question 33). The last intermediate step prior to doubling the dose would be to use an H₂RA at bedtime. This has sound short-term logic and is less expensive than adding a second dose of PPI. Short-term improvement in overnight pH control is seen when an over-the-counter dose of ranitidine (75 mg) is added at bedtime to omeprazole 20 mg before breakfast for 28 days. A study comparing omeprazole 20 mg plus ranitidine 150 mg at bedtime to omeprazole 20 mg twice daily favored the PPI twice daily for overall (including nocturnal) pH control. One study examined the effect of ranitidine 150 mg HS compared to placebo in patients on once-daily PPI who had continued nighttime symptoms. No difference was seen in overall efficacy between the 2 groups. Therefore I only use this approach when continued symptoms are intermittent and/or the patient can clearly delineate when they are going to have nighttime symptoms. The "prn" use of H₂ receptor antagonists (H₂RAs) seems to be best in this clinical scenario.

The optimal approach to the patient with typical or atypical symptoms suspected due to GERD who is still symptomatic on twice daily PPI is to perform a thorough and careful

Table 23-1
Intrasubject Variability in Intragastric pH Control: Esomeprazole Versus Other Proton Pump Inhibitors

Comparison *(n = 34)*	Favored comparator (% of patients with a higher percentage of time pH > 4.0)
Esomeprazole 40 mg vs pantoprazole 40 mg	Esomeprazole (88)
Esomeprazole 40 mg vs rabeprazole 20 mg	Esomeprazole (79)
Esomeprazole 40 mg vs omeprazole 20 mg	Esomeprazole (74)
Esomeprazole 40 mg vs lansoprazole 30 mg	Esomeprazole (71)

evaluation to determine if reflux is responsible. This often involves multiple interventions including determining whether the patient had GERD in the first place. In our practice, the evaluation includes a careful history of PPI compliance and dose timing. Despite continued teaching of the importance of dosing PPIs prior to a meal, this is often ignored. When omeprazole IR is prescribed, many completely disregard meal timing. Although bedtime administration of this drug is reasonable, it is not clear that it can be taken anytime of day. I do not advocate the empiric use of H_2RA at bedtime, nor addition of a prokinetic agent unless nocturnal reflux and/or erosive esophagitis has been documented. In my experience the overall likelihood of success is low when H_2RA is used empirically, and prolonged pH more valuable. We perform endoscopy if one has not been done or carefully reported. This is granted of low yield from the standpoint of finding erosive esophagitis, but may document the presence of Barrett's, a rare but other structural cause for symptoms (large hernia, ulcer), and allow for accurate placement of a telemetry pH capsule. In addition, there is the still to be defined value of a negative endoscopy for the patient and indeed the treating physician. Barium studies are rarely performed except in the presence of dysphagia, in which case we would suspect achalasia.

Bibliography

Katz PO. GERD symptoms on antisecretory therapy: acid, non-acid or no GERD. *Rev Gastroenterol Disord.* 2006;6(3):136-145.

WHAT ARE THE SHORT- AND LONG-TERM RISKS OF PROTON PUMP INHIBITOR THERAPY? ARE ANY RISKS OF CLINICAL IMPORTANCE?

These agents are among the safest used in medicine (Figure 24-1). Headache, abdominal pain, and diarrhea are the most common side effects and these are seen in no greater frequency than placebo in clinical trials. Concerns regarding long-term acid suppression and an increase in gastric carcinoid tumors have not been seen. Fundic gland polyps are seen in a small percentage of patients on proton pump inhibitor (PPI); however, to date the polys have universally been shown to have benign histology and are not a risk for "bad" outcomes. Though careful observational and case-control studies are needed, I do not adjust or stop PPIs in patients with fundic gland polyps *unless* the patient requests an alternative approach. I do not at present do follow-up endoscopy to monitor fundic gland polyps unless symptoms relapse or patients are in surveillance for Barrett's esophagus. B12 malabsorption has been suggested as a concern but has not been documented in any well-done studies outside of patients with multiple endocrine neoplasias. I do not check B12 levels or give B12 shots to any patients.

Concern is sometimes raised regarding a decrease in iron absorption on PPIs as patients with achlorhydria may not absorb iron as efficiently. To date, there is no documentation in the literature of any adverse effect of PPIs on iron supplementation, if it is even needed.

There is a theoretical interaction between all PPIs and warfarin and the package inserts warn that patients on concomitant PPIs and anticoagulation with warfarin should have careful monitoring of INR and prothrombin time to avoid problems. I have not encountered any issue in practice but we need to be vigilant. A theoretic decrease in theophylline efficacy exists but I have not seen it in my practice. PPIs may effect drugs whose pKa is

Figure 24-1. Long-term tolerability of PPIs. (Reprinted from Klinkenberg-Knol EC, Nelis F, Dent J, Snel P, Mitchell B, Prichard P, Lloyd D, Hacu N, Frame MH, Roman J, Walan A; Long-Term Study Group. Long-term omeprazole treatment in resistant gastroesophageal reflux disease: efficacy, safety, and influence on gastric mucosa. *Gastroenterology.* 2000;118:661-669, with permission from Elsevier.)

Data Demonstrating the Long-Term Tolerability of PPIs

- Klinkenberg-Knol et al. (2000)
  - 230 patients with severe erosive esophagitis treated with ≥ 20 mg omeprazole daily for a mean of 6.5 years (range: 1.1 to 11 years)
  - No gastric dysplasia or neoplasia were observed
  - Low incidence of gastric corpus mucosal atrophy
    - 4.7% in H. pylori-positive patients
    - 0.7% in H. pylori-negative patients
  - Low incidence of gastric corpus intestinal atrophy
    - Mild in 3 H. pylori-positive patients at last biopsy

Table 24-1

Risk of Hip Fracture Associated with Increasing Cumulative Duration of Proton Pump Inhibitor Therapy

Cumulative Proton Pump Inhibitor Therapy Duration (years)

	1	2	3	4
Crude	1.43 (1.35-1.52)	1.84 (1.67-2.01)	2.10 (1.91-2.35)	2.17 (1.93-2.45)
Adjusted†	1.22 (1.15-1.30)	1.41 (1.28-1.56)	1.54 (1.37-1.73)	1.59 (1.39-1.80)

Data are OR (95% CI).* CI, confidence interval; OR, odds ratio.
*The ORs are from the conditional logistic regression model matched by year of birth, sex, and both calendar period and duration of follow up before the index date, and included a quadratic term for duration of proton pump inhibitor therapy in years (P < .001 for the test of significance for the quadratic term).
†Adjusted for matching variables and all potential confounders.

Reprinted from Yang YX, Lewis JD, Epstein S, Metz DC. Long-term proton pump inhibitor therapy and risk of hip fracture. *JAMA.* 2006;296:2947-2953, with permission from the American Medical Association.

such that acid is required for their optimal efficacy. Iron (mentioned above) is one. The antifungal drugs—ketoconazole and itraconazole—may be affected but not fluconazole. PPIs may alter digoxin levels in theory, but I have not encountered problems (Table 24-1).

Several other areas of concern have been raised. An increased odds ratio of pneumonia has been reported in one study of patients on PPI (and H$_2$ receptor antagonists [H$_2$RAs]) compared to those not using the agent. The odds ratio for pneumonia was 1.8 compared

Table 24-2

Risk of Hip Fracture Associated With Increasing Daily Dosages of Proton Pump Inhibitor and Histamine 2 Receptor Antagonist Therapies

No. (%) of Participants OR (95% CI)*	Cases	Controls	Crude	Adjusted†
>1 year of H2RA ≤1.75 average daily dose	345 (2.53)	2189 (1.61)	1.66 (1.48-1.86)	1.23 (1.09-1.40)
>1.75 average daily dose	387 (2.84)	2289 (1.68)	1.78 (1.60-1.99)	1.30 (1.16-1.46)
>1 year of PPI ≤1.75 average daily dose	534 (3.94)	3228 (2.38)	1.77 (1.61-1.95)	1.40 (1.26-1.54)
≥1.75 average daily dose	37 (.027)	123(0.09)	3.18 (2.20-4.60)	2.65 (1.80-3.90)

CI, confidence interval; H2RA, histamine 2 receptor antagonist; OR, odds ratio; PPI, proton pump inhibitor.
*The ORs are from a conditional logistic regression model matched by year of birth, sex, and both calendar period and duration of follow up before the index date.
†Adjusted for matching variables and all potential confounders.

Reprinted from Yang YX, Lewis JD, Epstein S, Metz DC. Long-term proton pump inhibitor therapy and risk of hip fracture. *JAMA.* 2006;296:2947-2953, with permission from the American Medical Association.

Table 24-3

Potential Outcomes of Increased Intragastric pH on Drug Absorption

Absorption Increased (1)	Absorption Decreased
• Aspirin	• Ketoconazole (2)
• Benzylpenicillin	• Itraconazole (2)
• Nifedipine	
• Midazolam	
• Furosemide	• Indomethacin (1)
• Digoxin	• Iron supplements (1)

(1) Unlikely clinical importance, but watch carefully.
(2) May be clinically important.

to those not on PPI. The methodology of this study has been criticized and clinical observations do not support an increase in pneumonia. Several recent case-control studies have reported an increase in the prevalence of *Clostridium difficile* infection in patients on PPIs. Odds ratios from 1.3 to 5.1 for infection have been reported. These case-control studies have not been substantiated in direct observational studies, nor is the mechanism for this increase clear. Most importantly, the overall incidence of C. *difficile* infection in the general population is quite low, so any increase, even if it is "real," is unlikely to be a major clinical problem. Several caveats. Association does not prove causality and case-control studies, even when carefully designed, are limited in that they use data that are usually not systematically collected. Nevertheless, clinicians should be aware of the potential for C. *difficile* infection in patients on PPI, particularly if they require antibiotics, and in patients who are immunosuppressed, hospitalized, or in chronic care facilities.

A recent case-control study also found an increase in the odds ratio of hip fractures in patients on PPI, particularly those who used the drugs long term and in higher doses. The authors report that they accounted for multiple confounders, including the severity and number of comorbid conditions in the comparator groups (Tables 24-2 and 24-3). This association is plausible as PPI may affect calcium absorption. If confirmed, these data may affect the way we use PPIs long term, particularly in patients at risk for fracture. I am currently not changing my practice but am reminding patients at risk to discuss preventative measures with their primary care providers.

It is important to note that in a large observational study ($N = 230$) in which patients were followed while on continuous PPI, in doses of 20 to 160 mg/day of omeprazole for up to 11 continuous years, few if any long-term side effects were seen, including those discussed above.

A 42-Year-Old Man Who Does Not Use Tobacco or Alcohol but Has Chronic Reflux Presents for Evaluation and Wants to Know If He Is at Risk for Esophageal Cancer. What Do I Tell Him? Does His Risk Change if His Symptoms Are Effectively Relieved With PPI Therapy?

Esophageal adenocarcinoma has increased substantially over the past several decades and is now the fastest rising cancer among white males in the United States. Although the risk factors of long duration, higher frequency, and perhaps increased severity of nocturnal reflux symptoms are associated with an increased risk of developing adeno-carcinoma (Figures 25-1 and 25-2), the prevailing clinical opinion is that patients with chronic gastroesophageal reflux disease are not at risk for the development of esophageal adenocarcinoma unless they have underlying intestinal metaplasia (Barrett's esophagus) (Figure 25-3). A large case-control study showed that the risk for cancer increased with increasing prevalence of heartburn and was higher in patients with symptoms greater than 3 times a week. This same study showed an increase in the prevalence of esophageal cancer in patients with nocturnal symptoms. Identification of which Barrett's patients are

Figure 25-1. GERD symptom duration and frequency in esophageal adenocarcinoma. (Reprinted from Lagergren J, Bergstrom R, Lindgren A, Nyren O. Symptomatic gastroesophageal reflux as a risk factor for esophageal adenocarcinoma. *N Engl J Med.* 1999;340:825-831, with permission from Massachusetts Medical Society.)

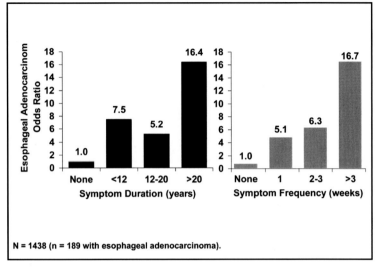

N = 1438 (n = 189 with esophageal adenocarcinoma).

Figure 25-2. Reflux symptoms duration and cancer risk. (Reprinted from Lagergren J, Bergstrom R, Lindgren A, Nyren O. Symptomatic gastroesophageal reflux as a risk factor for esophageal adenocarcinoma. *N Engl J Med.* 1999;340:825-831, with permission from Massachusetts Medical Society.)

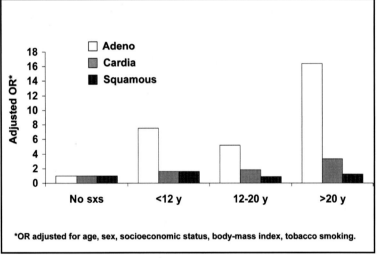

*OR adjusted for age, sex, socioeconomic status, body-mass index, tobacco smoking.

at risk is difficult. The presence of a large hiatal hernia (greater than 3 to 5 cm), a body mass index greater than 30 kg/m^2 and the presence of dysplasia on initial endoscopy have been identified as additional risks (Figure 25-4, Table 25-1). It should be noted importantly that recent epidemiologic studies have estimated the risk of developing adenocarcinoma from Barrett's to be extremely low (0.4% to 0.5% per patient year), reinforcing that the individual patient is actually of low risk. These numbers have important implications for management. Although tobacco and/or alcohol use has been shown to be associated with the development of squamous cell cancer of the esophagus, they have not been directly linked to the development of adenocarcinoma (Figure 25-5). As such, there is no real way to assess this 42-year-old man's risk for esophageal cancer in the absence of a screening endoscopy to determine if he has Barrett's esophagus. Adenocarcinoma of the esophagus is more prevalent in Caucasian men and squamous cell cancer of the esophagus is more

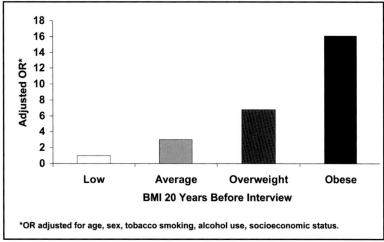

Figure 25-3. Prevalence of probable Barrett's esophagus relative to GERD symptom duration. (Reprinted from Lieberman DA, Oehlke M, Helfand M. Risk factors for Barrett's esophagus in community-based practice. GORGE constortium. Gastroenterology Outcomes Research Group in Endoscopy. *Am J Gastroenterol.* 1997;92:1293-1297, with permission from Elsevier.)

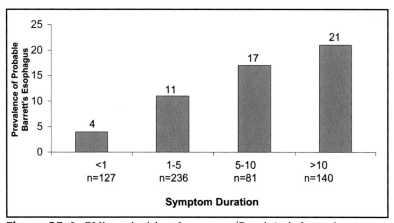

Figure 25-4. BMI and risk of cancer. (Reprinted from Lagergren J, Bergstrom R, Nyren O. Association between body mass and adenocarcinoma of the esophagus and gastric cardia. *Ann Intern Med.* 1999;130:883-890, with permission from American College of Physicians–American Society of Internal Medicine.)

prevalent in African Americans and in smokers and users of alcohol. Overall, however, the incidence of squamous cell cancer of the esophagus is decreasing and there is little discussion or concern about screening for this disease. Although he will benefit from the standpoint of improved quality of life, if his symptoms are effectively relieved with proton pump inhibitor therapy, there is little evidence that the latter will change his risk of developing esophageal cancer. I would reinforce that he should have a screening endoscopy for the best reassurance.

Figure 25-5. Reflux symptoms frequency and cancer risk. (Reprinted from Lagergren J, Bergstrom R, Lindgren A, Nyren O. Symptomatic gastroesophageal reflux as a risk factor for esophageal adenocarcinoma. *N Engl J Med.* 1999;340:825-831, with permission from Massachusetts Medical Society.)

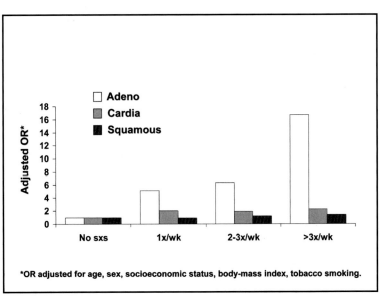

*OR adjusted for age, sex, socioeconomic status, body-mass index, tobacco smoking.

Table 25-1

Risk Factors for Esophageal Adenocarcinoma

- Gender
- Ethnicity
- Age
- Dysplasia
- Barrett's length
- Hiatal hernia length

Weston AP, Bard AS, Hassanein RS: Prospective multivariate analysis of factors predictive of complete regression of Barrett's esophagus. *Am J Gastroenterol.* 1999;94:3413-3419.
Reid BJ, Levine DS, Longton G, Blount PL, Rabinovitch PS. Predictors of progression to cancer in Barrett's esophagus: baseline histology and flow cytometry identify low- and high-risk patient subsets. *Am J Gastroenterol.* 2000;95(7):1669-1676.

Bibliography

El-Serag HB, Aguirre TV, Davis S, et al. Proton pump inhibitors are associated with reduced incidence of dysplasia in Barrett's esophagus. *Am J Gastroenterol.* 2004;99(10):1877-1883.
Hillman LC, Charagakis L, Shadbolt B, et al. Proton-pump inhibitor therapy and the development of dysplasia in patients with Barrett's oesophagus. *Med J Aust.* 2004;180(9):387-391.
Leedham S, Jankowski J. The evidence base of proton pump inhibitor chemopreventive agents in Barrett's esophagus—the good, the bad and the flawed! *Am J Gastroenterol.* 2007;102(1):21-23.

WHO IS AT RISK FOR BARRETT'S ESOPHAGUS? DO AFRICAN AMERICANS NEED TO WORRY ABOUT BARRETT'S ESOPHAGUS?

The current working definition, as defined by the American College of Gastroenterology (ACG) guidelines, is a change in the esophageal epithelium of any length that can be recognized during endoscopy and is confirmed by biopsy to have intestinal metaplasia. The working definition excludes intestinal metaplasia of the cardia as part of the definition of Barrett's esophagus. The current definition seeks to eliminate the concept of long or short segment Barrett's. Whether patients with GERD should be screened for Barrett's esophagus is debated, as it has been difficult to demonstrate that screening alters the natural history of the disease. Although the most recent ACG guidelines address in some detail surveillance of patients with endoscopically confirmed Barrett's esophagus (see below), issues relating to screening are not as carefully discussed. It is clearly logical to suggest that early identification of Barrett's esophagus would have the potential to identify those at risk and, perhaps, better stratify those who are candidates for long-term surveillance. Unfortunately, no prospective studies support this logic. Although the guidelines suggest screening patients over the age of 50 who are Caucasian, male, and have had symptoms for more than 5 to 10 years, this addresses only the highest-risk group. As recent data suggest, as many as 25% of asymptomatic individuals undergoing upper endoscopy at the time of colorectal screening have Barrett's. These data have been reproduced in at least two additional studies, one of which also showed a prevalence of Barrett's in 8.1% of women presenting for colonoscopy with minimal to no reflux symptoms. As such, there is some argument for widespread screening even in minimally or asymptomatic people. Although at present the economics of screening and surveying patients with Barrett's is

---

Table 26-1
Barrett's Esophagus Risk Factors

- Age >50 years
- White men
- GERD symptoms
  - Early age of onset
  - Longer duration

---

extremely expensive, cost-modeling studies suggest that it may be most cost effective to screen and survey only those with dysplasia on initial biopsy (Table 26-1).

Many risk factors have been evaluated as important in determining risk of Barrett's esophagus. Unfortunately, no classic picture emerges. The disease typically occurs in patients over the age of 40 with a long history of GERD. Cases are less frequently seen in younger people including the pediatric age group. The disease is 1.5 to 4.0 times more frequent in men and is more common in Caucasians than African Americans, Hispanics, and Asians in the United States. Other risk factors include a long duration of GERD symptoms and development of reflux at an early age (prior to age 35). Controversial risk factors include nocturnal reflux symptoms, obesity, and smoking. The importance of length of GERD symptoms as a risk for Barrett's is highlighted in the study by Lieberman and colleagues, who reviewed a large endoscopic database and found that the frequency of suspected Barrett's approached 20% when symptoms were present for greater than 10 years before the index endoscopy.

Unfortunately, there is not one person with GERD who can be presumed as having zero risk. Although it is nice to tell someone the risk is low, the only way to know if it is zero is to look, biopsy when necessary, and follow the patient.

Bibliography

Cameron AJ, Lomboy CT. Barrett's esophagus: age, prevalence, and extent of columnar epithelium. *Gastroenterology.* 1992;103:1241-1245.

Lieberman DA, Oehlke M, Helfand M. Risk factors for Barrett's esophagus in community based practice. GORGE consortium. Gastroenterology Outcomes Research Group in Endoscopy. *Am J Gastroenterol.* 1997;92:1293-1297.

Sampliner RE. Practice Parameters Committee of the American College of Gastroenterology. Updated guidelines for the diagnosis, surveillance, and therapy of Barrett's esophagus. *Am J Gastroenterol.* 2002;97:1888-1895.

SHOULD PATIENTS BE SCREENED FOR BARRETT'S? ARE THERE PATIENTS WHO NEED NOT BE SCREENED?

The current working definition for Barrett's esophagus as defined by the American College of Gastroenterology (ACG) guidelines is a change in the esophageal epithelium of any length that can be recognized during endoscopy and is confirmed by biopsy to have intestinal metaplasia. The working definition excludes intestinal metaplasia of the cardia as part of the definition of Barrett's esophagus. The current definition seeks to eliminate the concept of long or short segment Barrett's. Whether patients with GERD should be screened for Barrett's esophagus is debated, as it has been difficult to demonstrate that screening alters the natural history of the disease. Although the most recent ACG guidelines address in some detail surveillance of patients with endoscopically confirmed Barrett's esophagus (see below), issues relating to screening are not as carefully discussed. It is clearly logical to suggest that early identification of Barrett's esophagus would have the potential to identify those at risk and, perhaps, better stratify those who are candidates for long-term surveillance. Unfortunately, no prospective studies support this logic. Although the guidelines suggest screening patients over the age of 50 who are Caucasian, male, and have had symptoms for more than 5 to 10 years, this addresses only the highest-risk group. As recent data suggest, as many as 25% of asymptomatic individuals undergoing upper endoscopy at the time of colorectal screening have Barrett's. These data have been reproduced in at least two additional studies, one of which also showed a prevalence of Barrett's in 8.1% of women presenting for colonoscopy with minimal to no reflux symptoms. As such, there is some argument for widespread screening even in minimally or asymptomatic people. Although at present the economics of screening and surveying patients with Barrett's is extremely expensive, cost-modeling studies suggest that it may be most cost effective to screen and survey only those with dysplasia on initial biopsy.

If the patient is to be screened, it is best to do so after a trial of antisecretory therapy to eliminate and confounding erosive esophagitis and make landmarks easier to discern. Even in this setting, the endoscopist's dilemma is in the interpretation of which anatomic landmarks actually distinguish the end of the tubular esophagus from the gastric cardia. As it is crucial to biopsy only areas of columnar-appearing mucosa extending proximal to the gastroesophageal junction, this identification is clearly important. Staining with Lugol's iodine, toluidine blue, indigo carmine, and methylene blue have been suggested as methods to help recognize the junction; however, these methods have not obtained widespread use and are currently not the standard of practice. It seems reasonable to define the end of the tubular esophagus as the point at the top of the gastric folds seen in a decompressed stomach and esophagus. Columnar epithelium above this anatomic landmark should be considered for biopsy, whereas tissue below this landmark should not undergo biopsy because most investigators in the field believe that intestinal metaplasia of the gastric cardia is a condition more commonly associated with *Helicobacter pylori* infection, not GERD, and does not seem to progress to cancer. Appropriate histopathologic diagnosis therefore depends upon this approach.

In reality, no GERD patient is without some risk for developing Barrett's and as such all patients with chronic symptoms are candidates for screening. The decision to do so must take into account access, cost to the patient, and implications of making a diagnosis of Barrett's.

Bibliography

Sampliner RE. Practice Parameters Committee of the American College of Gastroenterology. Updated guidelines for the diagnosis, surveillance, and therapy of Barrett's esophagus. *Am J Gastroenterol*. 2002;97(8):1888-1895.

ARE THE PHARMACOLOGIC OPTIONS FOR BARRETT'S DIFFERENT FROM GERD? HAVE PPIS BEEN SHOWN TO HAVE ANY EFFECT ON BARRETT'S (EITHER PREVENTION OR THERAPY)?

The primary controversy in Barrett's esophagus relates to what form of therapy is "best" and, more importantly, whether any therapy results in the regression of abnormal epithelium or more importantly reduces the rate of progression to dysplasia and/or adenocarcinoma. The current standard of practice suggests that patients with Barrett's should be treated in similar fashion to patients with typical GERD, that is with antisecretory agents as needed to provide complete symptom relief. The most recent American College of Gastroenterology (ACG) guidelines point out correctly that there are no prospective studies that support that any alternative approach to treatment, either high-dose acid suppression or antireflux surgery, can reduce the risk of dysplasia or esophageal adenocarcinoma. However, there are several areas of concern and several lines of evidence that suggest that simply controlling symptoms is inadequate. Several studies have documented that despite the elimination of symptoms, a majority of patients with Barrett's esophagus will continue to have abnormal esophageal acid exposure, especially at night. Therefore, elimination of symptoms does not guarantee elimination of reflux. If one believes that the maintenance of normal epithelial differentiation and proliferation is essential to cancer chemoprevention and acid is the primary initiator of epithelial differentiation and proliferation, then elimination of all acid would be an important goal. Support for this comes from elegant studies in which biopsy specimens from patients with Barrett's and normal esophagi were exposed to acid in cell culture (continuously

Figure 28-1. Retrospective study showing a decrease in dysplasia in patients on proton pump inhibitors. (Reprinted from El-Serag HB, Aguirre TV, Davis S, et al. Proton pump inhibitors are associated with reduced incidence of dysplasia in Barrett's esophagus. *Am J Gastroenterol.* 2004;99[10]:1877-1883, with permission from Blackwell Publishing.)

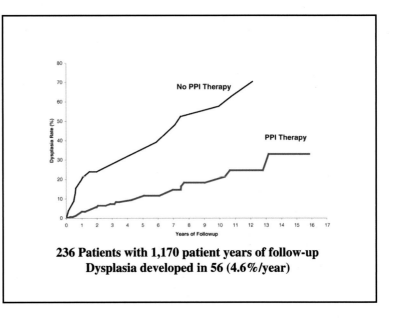

236 Patients with 1,170 patient years of follow-up
Dysplasia developed in 56 (4.6%/year)

at pH 3.5 or to 1-hour pulses) and then compared with tissue exposed to pH of 7 for up to 24 hours. Differentiation was quantified by villin expression and proliferation by the measurement of proliferating cell nuclear antigen (PCNA) expression. The study showed that villin protein was expressed in 50% and 83% of specimens after 6 and 24 hours of continuous acid exposure, compared to 25% at baseline with no increase in villin in cells exposed to a neutral pH. PCNA expression was higher for all samples, regardless of pH, compared with normal esophageal specimens. Acid pulse was found to cause the greatest increase in PCNA expression, whereas continuous acid resulted in decreased proliferation compared with a neutral pH, suggested to be due to cell death. Reduction of esophageal acid exposure reduced PCNA expression to a greater degree than those who still were abnormal despite being asymptomatic.

Despite these intermediate marker studies, clinical trials examining the effect of proton pump inhibitors on regression of Barrett's mucosa have failed to demonstrate significant decrease in Barrett's length in multiple studies. Although some overgrowth of squamous "islands" can be demonstrated, except for short segments, disappearance of Barrett's mucosa is unlikely with proton pump inhibitors.

A recent study provides the first important evidence that proton pump inhibitors may indeed slow the development of dysplasia in patients with Barrett's esophagus (Figure 28-1). The authors reviewed the database of a single endoscopist in a VA (Veterans Administration) hospital over a 20-year period (1981 through 2000), with a single pathologist using standard criteria to diagnose Barrett's esophagus and dysplasia. Pharmacy records were reviewed in both computerized and research files and patients on proton pump inhibitors, H_2 receptor antagonists, or no antisecretory therapy were reviewed for the development of dysplasia after the diagnosis of Barrett's was made. In the follow-up period, 56 patients developed dysplasia (1170 patient years of follow up) with an annual incidence of 4.7%. Fourteen of 56 developed high-grade dysplasia. A multivariate analysis in the use of proton pump inhibitors after a Barrett's esophagus diagnosis was associated with a reduced risk of dysplasia (hazard ratio 0.25, 95% CI 0.13 to 0.17), $P < .001$ compared to H_2 receptor antagonists or no therapy. These results represent the first evidence of delay in progression of Barrett's in patients on proton pump inhibitors (PPIs). Unfortunately, the study is not of sufficient size or length to assess the impact on the development of cancer, nor were the records able to assess the PPI dose and/or compliance.

Therefore, a case can be made for the use of proton pump inhibitors as the antisecretory therapy of choice and a reasonable suggestion that high dose or aggressive antisecretory therapy may be of value. If a clinician takes this approach, it is important to remember that normalization of esophageal acid exposure in Barrett's esophagus is difficult and is not always achieved with twice-daily dosing of PPIs. In fact, "normalization" of esophageal acid exposure is seen in only 80% to 85% of patients on PPI twice daily. As such, if normalization of acid control is desired, prolonged pH monitoring may be needed and can be done with the catheter-free Bravo device at the time of surveillance. This aggressive approach is controversial and has not been tested. Many will use a middle ground approach and treat with twice-daily dosing and leave the patient on this indefinitely if they are asymptomatic.

My personal practice is to review the options with the patient and make decisions together. In fact, most of my patients are on twice-daily PPI and have undergone pH testing to document that esophageal acid control has normalized. I follow them closely with endoscopic surveillance, which in my opinion is the "right" strategy for all patients with Barrett's regardless of therapy.

Bibliography

El-Serag HB, Aguirre TV, Davis S, et al. Proton pump inhibitors are associated with reduced incidence of dysplasia in Barrett's esophagus. *Am J Gastroenterol.* 2004;99(10):1877-1883.

Ouatu-Lascar R, Fitzgerald RC, Triadafilopoulos G. Differentiation and proliferation in Barrett's esophagus and the effects of acid suppression. *Gastroenterology.* 1999;117(2):327-335.

MR. SMITH HAS NO REFLUX SYMPTOMS BUT UNDERWENT UPPER ENDOSCOPY AS PART OF A CELIAC SPRUE EVALUATION. HE WAS FOUND TO HAVE A 5-MM SEGMENT OF COLUMNAR-LINED ESOPHAGUS WITHOUT NODULARITY. BIOPSIES SHOWED INTESTINAL METAPLASIA BUT NO DYSPLASIA. WHAT IS THE APPROPRIATE FOLLOW-UP?

Based on the current definition proposed by the American College of Gastroenterology guidelines and the American Gastroenterological Association Chicago Workshop, this patient has Barrett's esophagus. This working definition using displacement of the squamocolumnar junction proximal to the gastroesophageal junction with the presence of intestinal metaplasia on biopsy allows us to standardize our discussions. The entity of Barrett's esophagus has evolved over the past several decades to now include segments of columnar-lined esophagus with intestinal metaplasia that are less than 2 to 3 cm in length and are today still referred to as short-segment Barrett's esophagus (SSBE). The keys for the endoscopist are to differentiate a columnar-lined esophagus, which should be biopsied from an irregular Z line, and to avoid biopsy of the gastric cardia, as it is important clinically in that the so-called short-segment Barrett's esophagus is a lesion with a malignant risk, whereas intestinal metaplasia of the gastric cardia probably is not. Today, we do that by using endoscopic landmarks, identifying the top of the gastric folds, avoiding overinflation during endoscopy. The addition of chromoendoscopic techniques with methylene blue has been used but has produced inconsistent results and is not routinely recommended in the endoscopy laboratory. Similarly, the use of cytokeratin staining has also been inconsistent in results, therefore limiting its utility in routine clinical practice.

Although the natural history of short-segment Barrett's esophagus is not clearly understood, there is little doubt that esophageal adenocarcinoma can develop in these patients; and although it may be seen in lower frequency than in long-segment Barrett's esophagus, there is little chance in current practice to avoid putting these patients into a surveillance program. As such, the diagnosis of short-segment Barrett's likely commits the patient to a surveillance program identical to that of long-segment Barrett's (see Question 30). Based on current available data, surveillance is not recommended by most experts for intestinal metaplasia of the gastric cardia. While we await further research and hopefully better risk stratification for patients with Barrett's esophagus, the patient in question would, in my practice, be offered surveillance.

Bibliography

Sampliner RE. Practice Parameters Committee of the American College of Gastroenterology. Updated guidelines for the diagnosis, surveillance, and therapy of Barrett's esophagus. *Am J Gastroenterol.* 2002;97(8):1888-1895.

Sharma P, McQuaid K, Dent J, et al. AGA Chicago Workshop. A critical view of the diagnosis and mangement of Barrett's esophagus: the AGA Chicago Workshop. *Gastroenterology.* 2004;127:310-330.

Spechler SJ, Zeroogian JM, Antonioli, DA, Wang HH, Goyal RK. Prevalence of metaplasia at the gastro-oesophageal junction. *Lancet.* 1994;344:1533-1536.

Weston AP, Krmpotich P, Makdisi WF, et al. Short segment Barrett's esophagus: clinical and histological features, associated with endoscopic findings, and association with gastric intestinal metaplasia. *Am J Gastroenterol.* 1996;91:981-986.

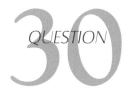

SHOULD ENDOSCOPIC SURVEILLANCE BE PERFORMED IN A PATIENT WITH BARRETT'S? IF SO, HOW?

There is little argument among clinicians that patients with Barrett's esophagus should be put in a surveillance program. Surveillance strategies are designed to detect premalignant or early malignant lesions so that death from cancer can be prevented. Though the incidence of esophageal adenocarcinoma is low, 0.3% to 0.5% per patient year, the lifetime incidence in a given patient may be as high as 10% to 11%, suggesting that surveillance might be beneficial.

Despite these data and the logic that early detection of high-grade dysplasia or intramucosal cancer would result in prolonged survival, prospective data supporting the effectiveness of on going surveillance for patients with Barrett's esophagus is lacking. Many have argued that only a small percentage of patients with Barrett's esophagus die of adenocarcinoma, that patients with Barrett's have the same life expectancy as those without, and that surveillance has little impact on this ultimate outcome. Cost-modeling studies argue against the use of surveillance in patients who have no dysplasia on initial biopsy. Contrasting data from retrospective surgical series strongly suggest that adenocarcinoma discovered on surveillance endoscopy have earlier stages and better 2-year survival than patients who present with cancer at the initial endoscopy. Cancers found on a surveillance endoscopy have been demonstrated to have a greater 5-year survival than cancers found when discovered when the patient presents with symptoms of dysphagia. Two cohort studies have documented earlier stage disease and improved survival in patients with a prior endoscopic diagnosis of Barrett's, suggesting that endoscopy offers the opportunity for intervening in earlier stage disease. Thus, the guidelines from the American College of Gastroenterology (ACG) and current standard of care are to perform surveillance endoscopy at a defined interval, depending on the degree of dysplasia on initial screening (Figure 30-1). The intervals suggested are based on a compilation of

Figure 30-1. Recommended surveillance of Barrett's esophagus. (Reprinted from Sampliner RE. Practice Parameters Committee of the American College of Gastroenterology. Updated guidelines for the diagnosis, surveillance, and therapy of Barrett's esophagus. *Am J Gastroenterol.* 2002;97[8]:1888-1895, with permission from Elsevier.)

Recommended Surveillance of BE

Dysplasia Grade	Cancer/n	Percent	Follow-up (years)	Proposed Follow-up Endoscopy
None	5/150	3	3.4-10	After 2 negative; every 2-3 years
LGD	8/45	18	1.5-4.3	Every 6 months x 2; then every year
HGD	21/61	34	0.2-4.5	Reconfirm; selective resection or endoscopy every 3 months

Figure 30-2. Surveillance of Barrett's esophagus: cost effectiveness. (Reprinted from Provenzale D, Kemp JA, Arora S, Wong JB. A guide for surveillance of patients with Barrett's esophagus. *Am J Gastroenterol.* 1994;89:670-680, with permission from Elsevier.)

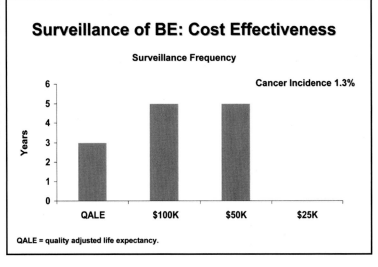

Surveillance of BE: Cost Effectiveness

QALE = quality adjusted life expectancy.

studies from a total of over 1600 patients followed for a mean of 2.9 to 7.3 years showing that the mean interval for progression to cancer is broad. Surveillance intervals in the guidelines are also balanced by cost-modeling studies, plotted against quality of life years saved (Figure 30-2).

There are two key issues. Dysplasia may be focal and, as such, diagnosis may be subject to sampling error. Therefore, the initial endoscopy should be repeated in approximately 1 year to rule out early dysplasia and to decrease sampling error. Careful attention to the suggested biopsy protocol is needed. Four-quadrant biopsies, every 1 to 2 cm with large capacity biopsy forceps, are recommended although there is some debate as to necessity to do this. As there is a greater risk of sampling error for high-grade dysplasia and adenocarcinoma, if large capacity biopsy forceps are not used, some suggest the sampling interval be as close as 1 cm apart so that more biopsies can be obtained. There is evidence that biopsy protocols are not routinely followed nor are landmarks adequately documented in clinical practice.

Current ACG guidelines recommend a 2- to 3-year interval between surveillance endoscopies in patients with no dysplasia after 2 endoscopic evaluations 1 year apart. A 5-year interval may make this practice more cost effective. If low-grade dysplasia is documented, then annual endoscopies should be performed until no dysplasia is found. Low-grade dysplasia is less likely to progress and often regresses. High-grade dysplasia presents the most critical dilemma and will be discussed subsequently.

At present, it is standard of practice in the United States to survey patients with Barrett's esophagus and hard to defend if it is not done. I follow the ACG guidelines in my practice, varying only when patients decline to follow. There are occasions when I will survey more frequently than recommended by guidelines, specifically in patients with very long segments (>5 cm). Although difficult to support based on current evidence, I believe those with longer segments are at higher risk for cancer development and usually survey them more frequently.

Bibliography

Sampliner RE. Practice Parameters Committee of the American College of Gastroenterology. Updated guidelines for the diagnosis, surveillance, and therapy of Barrett's esophagus. *Am J Gastroenterol*. 2002;97(8):1888-1895.

WHAT ARE THE MANAGEMENT OPTIONS FOR DYSPLASIA IN PATIENTS WITH BARRETT'S ESOPHAGUS, SPECIFICALLY HIGH-GRADE DYSPLASIA?

A dilemma for the clinician is how to manage a patient in whom high-grade dysplasia (HGD) is detected on biopsy. The first step in management is to confirm the diagnosis by review by an expert pathologist, as separating HGD from cancer can be difficult (Figure 31-1). Dysplasia should be classified as focal or diffuse. The controversy then revolves around the following. Should an immediate esophagectomy be performed, should the patient undergo intensive surveillance with esophagectomy performed only if cancer is discovered (so-called watchful waiting), or should ablation of the HGD be done?

Several studies have been reported on the frequency with which an unsuspected adenocarcinoma was found in patients operated on for HGD (Figure 31-2). When these studies are pooled, 80/184 patients (43%) are found to have a carcinoma. Unfortunately, these are small studies and the frequency of carcinoma varies from 0% to 73%. The outcome in these patients, of course, varies but these studies are often cited as evidence for performing esophagectomy early. However, the risk of leaving half of the patients with initially untreated cancer may outweigh the risk of the mortality from the operation, which varies based on hospital volume. In high-volume hospitals (>5 operations per year), mortality is lower (3.4%) than low-volume hospitals (17.3%). Overall, this high mortality should make the clinician pause before recommending esophagectomy and if chosen, the patient should go to a high-volume center.

Three studies have been reported recently that make a case for intensive surveillance rather than immediate esophagectomy in patients with HGD (Figure 31-2). One

Figure 31-1. Progression from intestinal metaplasia cancer is believed to move through the illustrated stages. What is not clear is the number, if any, who regress. In reality, many will progress slowly. (Reprinted from Ginsberg G, Fleischer DE. Esophageal tumors. In: *Sleisenger & Fordtran's Gastrointestinal and Liver Disease*, 7th ed; 2002:647-671, with permission from Elsevier.)

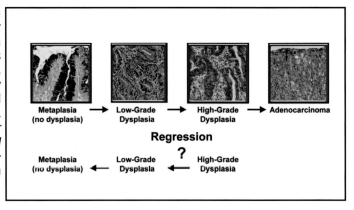

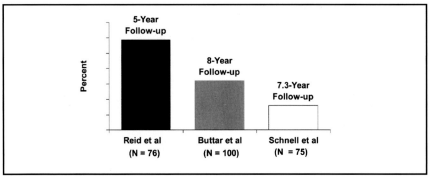

Figure 31-2. Progression of HGD to adenocarcinoma. (References: Reid BJ, Haggitt RC, Rubin CE, et al. Observer variation in the diagnosis of dysplasia in Barrett's esophagus. *Am J Gastroenterol*. 2000;95:1669-1676. Buttar NS, Wang KK, Sebo TJ, et al. Extent of high-grade dysplasia in Barrett's esophagus correlates with risk of adenocarcinoma. *Gastroenterology*. 2001;120:1630-1639. Schnell TG, Sontag SJ, Chejfec G. Long-term nonsurgical management of Barrett's esophagus with high-grade dysplasia. *Gastroenterology*. 2001;120:1607-1619.)

study reported on 50 patients. Fourteen had cancer on repeat biopsy and had immediate surgery (Figure 31-3). Seven with HGD underwent esophagectomy—none had cancer found. Subsequently, 29 patients were followed with periodic biopsies until a diagnosis of cancer was made. Seven subsequently developed cancer, all were resectable, none had metastasis to lymph nodes, and mortality was zero. The remaining patients were followed for a mean of 18 months and none developed cancer. A second study followed 72 patients with HGD for varying periods (mean follow up 7.3 years) and found 11 with adenocarcinoma, 11 of whom appeared to be cured with esophagectomy. The last patient was lost to follow up and did not have regular surveillance. Seventeen died of noncancer causes and still had HGD. The third found that about 30% of their patients with HGD progressed to cancer with mean follow up of 8 years. This group highlights the importance of focal versus diffuse HGD in the prevalence of cancer (see below). These studies highlight that many patients with HGD will not develop cancer over many years. The first study underscores the fact that a careful surveillance biopsy protocol can differentiate HGD from cancer. If HGD is to be followed, most recommend performing aggressive repeat biopsies every 3 months for the first year after discovery of HGD. If no

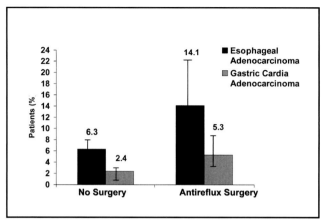

Figure 31-3. Antireflux surgery does not guarantee prevention of adenocarcinoma. (Reprinted from Ye W, Chow WH, Lagergren J, et al. Risk of adenocarcinomas of the esophagus and gastric cardia in patients with gastroesophageal reflux diseases and after antireflux surgery. *Gastroenterology.* 2001;121[6]:1286-1293, with permission from Elsevier.)

cancer is detected on 4 consecutive biopsies 3 months apart and the Barrett's is entirely flat (no elevated lesions), surveillance can be decreased to yearly with esophagectomy considered if cancer is found.

Patients unwilling to have or are poor candidates for esophagectomy and/or wish to "have something done" are candidates for ablative therapy. When considered, ablation can be performed with multipolar electrocautery, argon plasma coagulation, laser, or photodynamic therapy (PDT). The latter has been most widely reported. A photosensitizer absorbs light energy and transfers it to oxygen, resulting in tissue destruction. Four studies (N = 5 to 73) using different photosensitizers have ablated HGD in 88% to 100%. Unfortunately, side effects are not rare and include strictures, requiring dilatation in 15% to 30%, and severe chest pain. Intestinal metaplasia remains beneath the neosquamous epithelium and adenocarcinoma has been reported after PDT.

The only randomized trial, a multicenter study comparing PDT plus omeprazole 20 mg twice daily versus omeprazole alone, reported 3-year follow up showing a decreased number of patients evolving to cancer in the PDT-treated group compared to the control. Unfortunately, cancers did develop in the PDT group despite this treatment. The rate of cancer development in the omeprazole-alone group was higher than seen in any of 3 watchful waiting studies outlined above, underscoring the heterogenicity of these patients.

A new technology uses computer delivered radiofrequency (RFe) to ablate Barrett's tissue. A balloon is used to "size the esophagus" and to then apply the RFe. Early results are promising; complete ablation seems to be possible, and "buried Barrett's" has not been seen in early trials. Its place remains to be clarified but is exciting.

Patients with endoscopic mucosal irregularities or mass lesions demonstrating HGD can be considered for endoscopic mucosal resection (EMR) can be considered. EMR has been studied in observational studies as a treatment for macroscopically distinguishable lesions with HGD or intramucosal cancer (or limited tongues of Barrett's at the esophagogastric [EG] junction). Experts can successfully remove lesions at extremely low morbidity with extremely low or no perforations. A study from the Mayo Clinic compared intermediate outcomes (5-year follow up) of patients with Barrett's and intramucosal cancer who underwent combination endoscopic mucosal resection and PDT (N = 24) or esophagectomy (N = 64). This was a retrospective study and not randomized. The groups were comparable for tumor stage and segment length, but the patients undergoing mucosal resection and PDT were older and had more comorbid conditions. Elimination of intramucosal cancer was achieved in 83% of the EMR/PDT group. One eventually underwent esophagectomy and two died from unrelated causes. Strictures were seen in only 10% (substantially lower than the PDT literature in which stricture rates are as high as 30% to 35%). Additionally, operative mortality was low (1.6%). Though not completely comparable, there was no difference in the treatment arms. A recent publication reported "long-term" results in 100 patients undergoing EMR for HGD or early cancer. Ninety-nine were reported to have had a complete resection, no major complication, and no deaths. Recurrence was seen in 11% but all of these were cured on subsequent EMRs. These are experienced operators and well-selected patients. Nevertheless, the results are promising. Overall, EMR appears to be a promising option for management of macroscopic lesions with HGD and short segments of Barrett's. Whether it represents a cure or results in delay in progression to cancer remains to be seen.

Ultimately, the choice rests with the patient. This is the most difficult decision I encounter as there are no right answers. Fortunately, there is usually time to make a decision. I have one patient whom I have followed for 9 years with HGD who has just been found to have "progressed" to cancer. One can only wonder how long someone can live in equilibrium with his disease.

Bibliography

Ell C, May A, Pech O, et al. Curative endoscopic resection of early esophageal adenocarcinomas (Barrett's cancer). *Gastrointest Endosc.* 2007;65:3-10.

Ye W, Chow WH, Lagergren J, et al. Risk of adenocarcinomas of the esophagus and gastric cardia in patients with gastroesophageal reflux diseases and after antireflux surgery. *Gastroenterology.* 2001;121(6):1286-1293.

A Patient With Long-Standing GERD Does Not Wish to Take Long-Term Medical Therapy and Inquires About the Options for Treatment. He Wonders if There Is Something He Can Do Other Than Antireflux Surgery? Is There a Role for Endoscopic Therapy for GERD?

Millions of patients with GERD take proton pump inhibitors and safely obtain relief of reflux symptoms. However, many patients are hesitant to take daily medications and are even more hesitant to undergo antireflux surgery. Emerging options for such patients are the endoluminal GERD therapies that have evolved over the past several years, claiming efficacy comparable to antireflux surgery in GERD symptom relief. However, there has been a paucity of data to support that efficacy, even as more and more devices have been developed. Before adopting these treatments into any clinical practice, it is prudent to evaluate each therapy with respect to efficacy, safety, and durability. As of this writing, two therapies are still available for clinical use.

The two devices the Food and Drug Administration (FDA) approved for endoscopic treatment of GERD are gastric plication or suturing and radiofrequency energy. Bulking agents have been withdrawn and trials stopped. All were approved with limited uncontrolled data.

I do not currently offer endoscopic therapy in my practice as I do not find either of the available devices to be overwhelmingly successful. The newest plication device may hold promise, but I will wait for more data.

I have performed radiofrequency ablation and injection therapy and have no personal experience with sewing or plicator devices. I was underwhelmed by the radiofrequency energy results save one patient who was able to avoid proton pump inhibitors during pregnancy by undergoing the procedure prior to becoming pregnant. Her child is now about 5 years old and she needs little medication.

Evident from recent developments, interest in endoluminal GERD therapies continues, albeit somewhat attenuated from initial enthusiasm. It is equally clear that no single treatment has emerged as a safe and effective alternative to conventional medical or surgical therapy. The existing database of positive efficacy trials continues to consist largely of uncontrolled trials with somewhat convoluted designs and outcome measures that make comparisons with existing therapies difficult. Controlled trials continue to show either negative results or meager efficacy. Clearly, there is no evidence suggesting that these treatments have any role in the treatment of esophagitis or the complications of esophagitis, this remains to be the domain of antisecretory drugs and antireflux surgery. Similarly, endoluminal therapies should not be applied to patients with >2-cm hiatal hernias and no evidence exists for a role in the management of suspected supraesophageal manifestations of GERD. In addition, all existing controlled trials are short term (3 to 12 months) and have yet to demonstrate long-term benefit in terms of either symptom control or cost reduction. In brief, from an evidence-based perspective, no endoluminal GERD treatment has demonstrated meaningful efficacy, irrespective of regulatory approval.

The one consistent finding common to all of the reported endoluminal treatment trials is GERD symptom reduction. Although encouraging, this finding must be interpreted with caution. Placebo response rates for nonerosive reflux disease can be as high as 60% and, indeed, the observed sham response in the Enteryx trial was 53%. Similarly, using a reduction in proton pump inhibitor utilization as a primary end point is fraught with complexity. Many patients are overtreated with proton pump inhibitors and even trials switching among available proton pump inhibitors usually succeed in demonstrating dose reduction.

In conclusion, we need better data before endorsing the clinical use of endoluminal therapies for GERD. As it stands in early 2007, the available endoluminal GERD therapies are fewer than they were in 2005 and can still be characterized as having ill-defined benefit and clear potential risk. Patients with reflux disease interested in pursuing these treatments should be advised accordingly and ideally offered the opportunity to participate in well-designed trials to assess efficacy.

Bibliography

Montgomery M, Hakanson B, Ljungqvist O, et al. Twelve months' follow-up after treatment with the EndoCinch endoscopic technique for gastro-oesophageal reflux disease: a randomized, placebo-controlled study. *Scand J Gastroenterol.* 2006;41:1382-1389.

Rothstein R, Filipi C, Caca K, et al. Endoscopic full-thickness plication for the treatment of gastroesophageal reflux disease: a randomized, sham-controlled trial. *Gastroenterology.* 2006;131:704-712.

ARE THERE DIFFERENCES AMONG PPIs IN CLINICAL PRACTICE? SHOULD I EVER CONSIDER SWITCHING AMONG DIFFERENT PPIs FOR PATIENTS WHO FAIL TO RESPOND?

Careful examination of the many published pharmacodynamic studies reveals an often undiscussed but large interindividual and intraindividual variability in intragastric pH control with the various proton pump inhibitors (PPIs), either given once or even twice daily. This variability with twice-daily dosing is highlighted by a randomized crossover study in which healthy volunteers were given omeprazole 20 mg twice daily and lansoprazole 30 mg twice daily for 7 days separated by at least a 1-week washout period (Figure 33-1). Intragastric pH monitoring was performed on day 7. Subjects were asked to eat similar meals on each study day. The study results revealed a wide variability in 24-hour pH control with both drugs. In addition, there is intrasubject variability, with some patients responding well to omeprazole and not lansoprazole as well as the reverse seen in several subjects. Although this inter- and intrasubject variability may not be of clinical importance when evaluating large groups of patients, the variability in response to PPIs may have clinical implications when patients fail to respond to the first PPI prescribed.

An early study compared the intragastric pH profiles of single daily doses of omeprazole, lansoprazole, rabeprazole, and pantoprazole (20, 30, 20, 40 mg, respectively) in healthy subjects participating in clinical trials at a single institution. Intragastric pH studies from individuals who had taken each of the 4 PPIs before breakfast for 7 days under similar meal conditions and *Helicobactor pylori* status were reviewed. The percentage and number of hours of the 24-hour period in which the intragastric pH was greater than 4,

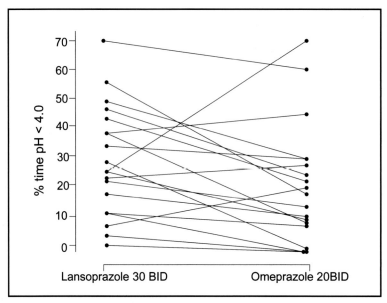

Figure 33-1. Study performed on 20 normal subjects showing marked variability of intragastric pH control among individuals even on twice-daily proton pump inhibition.

both upright and recumbent, was similar for all 4 PPIs. When the fifth PPI, esomeprazole, became available, separate studies were performed evaluating intragastric pH control of esomeprazole 40 mg once daily compared to each of the aforementioned PPIs at Food and Drug Administration (FDA)-approved doses for erosive esophagitis. Esomeprazole 40 mg demonstrated superior intragastric pH control compared to each of the other drugs.

Thus, a 5-arm randomized cross-over study in 24 *H. pylori*–negative patients with gastroesophageal reflux disease was performed. Esomeprazole 40 mg, rabeprazole 20 mg, lansoprazole 30 mg, pantoprazole 40 mg, and omeprazole 20 mg were compared. The drug was given 30 minutes before the breakfast meal for 5 days, with intragastric pH monitoring performed on day 5. This crossover study was completed with a 10- to 17-day washout period between treatments. The study demonstrated superiority for esomeprazole 40 mg compared to the other 4 PPIs in the number of hours and percentage of the 24-hour period in which the pH is greater than 4. In addition, the number of patients achieving this level of pH control for more than 12 hours was statistically superior for esomeprazole 40 mg compared to other PPIs. The clinical importance of the incremental difference in pH control cannot be ascertained from the study, but perhaps explain the difference in healing among esomeprazole and lansoprazole, omeprazole, and pantoprazole, particularly in patients with grade C and D erosive esophagitis.

A well-done, 6-arm crossover study comparing intragastric pH in *H. pylori*–negative healthy subjects on esomeprazole 20, 40, and 80 mg versus lansoprazole 15, 30, and 60 mg once daily before breakfast has also been reported in preliminary form. A washout period of at least 13 days was required between treatments to eliminate a carryover effect. A 24-hour intragastric pH monitoring study was performed on day 5, with results analyzed for median 24-hour intragastric pH. The study revealed that esomeprazole was superior to lansoprazole for each of the drug comparisons

Table 33-1

Intrasubject Variability in Intragastric pH Control: Esomeprazole Versus Other Proton Pump Inhibitors

Comparison (n = 34)	Favored comparator (% of patients with a higher percentage of time pH > 4.0)
Esomeprazole 40 mg vs pantoprazole 40 mg	Esomeprazole (88)
Esomeprazole 40 mg vs rabeprazole 20 mg	Esomeprazole (79)
Esomeprazole 40 mg vs omeprazole 20 mg	Esomeprazole (74)
Esomeprazole 40 mg vs lansoprazole 30 mg	Esomeprazole (71)

Table 33-2

Intragastric pH Control (Longer Time With pH > 4) With Esomeprazole Relative to Lansoprazole (n = 34)

Dose period	Higher values on esomeprazole (%)	Higher values on lansoprazole (%)	P value*
Eso 20 mg vs lanso 1.5 mg	76.5	23.5	<.01
Eso 20 mg vs lanso 30 mg	52.9	47.1	.9
Eso 40 mg vs lanso 30 mg	82.4	17.6	<.001
Eso 40 mg vs lanso 60 mg	85.3	14.7	<.001
Eso 80 mg vs lanso 60 mg	85.3	14.7	<.001

*Eso = esomeprazole; lanso = lansoprazole.

(20 versus 15 mg, 40 versus 60 mg, 80 versus 60 mg). It is important to note that the 24-hour intragastric pH control for the 80-mg once-daily does was 15.8 hours. This is numerically less than the 19.5 hours seen in a separate study assessing intragastric pH control on esomeprazole 40 mg bid, emphasizing improved efficacy of bid dosing when greater acid control is required. This study also examined interindividual variability in pH control, specifically the percentage of subjects that had superior pH control (time pH > 4) with esomeprazole relative to lansoprazole, and vice versa.

The 5-arm crossover study discussed above was analyzed for intersubject variability in intragastric pH control among the agents. Although esomeprazole was superior to the other PPIs in both percentage of patients and mean relative increase in percentage of time with the pH greater than 4 (Table 33-1), when evaluating these data, it is important to note that in some patients, another PPI will be superior to esomeprazole in 24-hour control of intragastric pH.

The 5-arm crossover study discussed above is outlined in Table 33-2.

In practice, switching PPIs makes sense only in the presence of side effects and cost differences. This is the only time I do it unless a pH study shows poor intragastric pH response on therapy.

Bibliography

Katz P, Miner P, Chen Y, Roach A, Sostek M. Effects of 5 marketed proton pump inhibitors on acid suppression relative to a range of pH thresholds. *Am J Gastroenterol.* 2004;99:S34.

Katz PO, Hatlebakk JG, Castell DO. Gastric acidity and acid breakthrough with twice-daily omeprazole or lansoprazole. *Aliment Pharmacol Ther.* 2000;14(6):709-714.

Miner P, Katz PO, Chen Y, Sostek M. Gastric acid control with esomeprazole, lansoprazole, omeprazole, pantoprazole, and rabeprazole: a five-way crossover study. *Am J Gastroenterol.* 2003;98:2616-2620.

IS THERE A ROLE FOR A COMBINATION OF PROTON PUMP INHIBITORS AND H_2 RECEPTOR ANTAGONISTS IN A PATIENT WITH GERD?

There is logic to adding an H_2 receptor antagonist (H_2RA) at bedtime to a proton pump inhibitor (PPI). H_2RAs given at bedtime in conjunction with a delayed-release PPI can augment overnight pH control. A single dose of an H_2RA (ranitidine 150 or 300 mg) given at bedtime in addition to a delayed-release PPI twice daily has been demonstrated to improve overnight pH control (Figure 34-1). The efficacy of H_2RAs is best with the first dose, maintains efficacy in the first week of therapy, and gives variability in pH control over time. Two papers highlight the important issues regarding long-term efficacy of this type of regimen.

A prospective study of 23 normal volunteers and 20 GERD patients studied at baseline with omeprazole 20 mg bid (before breakfast and dinner) for 2 weeks, followed by the addition of an H_2 receptor antagonist (ranitidine 300 mg qhs) at bedtime for 28 days. Patients were studied with prolonged ambulatory pH monitoring after days 1, 7, and 28 of continuous H_2RAs at bedtime.

The median time pH < 4 for overnight period was similar between patients and volunteers so were considered together. Four patterns of gastric pH response were found: The first group experienced a decreasing effect of baseline H_2RA over time (tolerance). The second consisted of 21% who exhibited a sustained response to H_2RA therapy (no tolerance). The third group had no nocturnal gastric acid breakthrough (NAB) on PPI twice daily and remained so when H_2RA was added. All in this group were *Helicobacter pylori positive*. The fourth group was marked by an unpredictable response (26%). This group showed variable outcome at different time points in their study.

Figure 34-1. Nocturnal acid breakthrough on bid PPIs. Effect of an H_2RA or PPI at bedtime given as a single dose. (Reprinted from Peghini PL, Katz PO, Castell DO. Ranitidine controls nocturnal gastric acid breakthrough on omeprazole: a controlled study in normal subjects. *Gastroenterology.* 1998;115:1335-1339, with permission from Elsevier.)

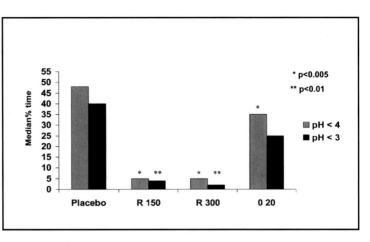

A retrospective review of prolonged ambulatory pH monitoring studies in patients comprised of 2 groups was also published. One had 60 patients taking either omeprazole 20 mg or lansoprazole 30 mg twice a day. The second had 45 patients on PPI twice a day (omeprazole 20 mg or lansoprazole 30 mg) plus an H_2 blocker at bedtime (ranitidine 300 mg, famotidine 40 mg, or nizatidine 300 mg) for greater than 28 days.

Twenty-seven percent of patients who were on H_2RAs at bedtime spent 100% of the recumbent period with intragastric pH greater than 4, 32% had greater than 90% of recumbent period above 4, and the remainder with lesser degrees of control. This was overall superior to PPI bid ($P < 0.001$). Eleven patients were tested on both regimens ($n = 11$). The median percentage time intragastric pH greater than 4 overnight increased from 54.6% without H_2RA to 96.5% with H_2RA at bedtime ($P = 0.001$). These studies come to different conclusions: the former concluding that tolerance develops quickly and there is no sustained control of intragastric pH over time with the addition of an H_2RA, and the latter that there is substantial benefit to the long-term use of these agents at bedtime. Careful evaluation of these studies suggests many similarities. In the study suggesting tolerance, 21% had a sustained response that is remarkably similar to the 27% in the other study. Both identify a substantial number of patients who have a sustained effect and many who do not. Both agree that achieving total acid control (100% time intragastric pH is greater than 4) is extremely difficult. It is thus reasonable to conclude that tolerance to H_2RAs at bedtime is real but relative and that a sustained response may be seen in some patients but not the majority. The studies underscore the importance of prolonged ambulatory pH monitoring as a means of documenting acid control and avoidance of using H_2RA HS empirically in difficult to treat patients.

A series of pharmacodynamic studies show a hierarchy of pH control starting with a PPI before breakfast, adding an H_2RA at bedtime, increasing to twice-daily PPI monotherapy, and finally adding an H_2RA at bedtime to twice-daily PPI therapy. No clinical trials demonstrate any symptom improvement with any of these regimens over a PPI alone, so it likely would be practical to add an H_2RA at bedtime to PPI therapy on an as-needed basis only for reasons of cost (Table 34-1).

I use an H_2RA at bedtime less frequently than in the past as many have already been tried on the combination before they are seen. Nighttime therapy with immediate-release

---

Table 34-1

Hierarchy of Intragastric pH Control

- PPI once a day
- PPI plus H2 HS (OTC probably OK)*
- PPI bid*
- PPI bid plus H2*

*These regimens have never been tested head to head in clinical trials!

---

omeprazole has changed my practice somewhat; *however,* each patient is treated individually and I *rarely* use an H$_2$RA or immediate-release omeprazole in refractory patients on an empiric basis. I almost always study the patient to determine if they still have nocturnal reflux!

Bibliography

Fackler WK, Ours TM, Vaezi MF, Richter JE. Long-term effect of H2RA therapy on nocturnal gastric acid breakthrough. *Gastroenterology.* 2002;122:625-632.

Peghini PL, Katz PO, Castell DO. Ranitidine controls nocturnal gastric acid breakthrough on omeprazole: a controlled study in normal subjects. *Gastroenterology.* 1998;115:1335-1339.

Xue S, Katz PO, Banerjee P, Tutuian R, Castell DO. Bedtime H2 blockers improve nocturnal gastric acid control in GERD patients on proton pump inhibitors. *Aliment Pharmacol Ther.* 2001;15:1351-1356.

What Is Nocturnal Acid Breakthrough, and What Is Its Clinical Importance? Is Zegerid Really Any More Effective in This Group?

This controversial and misunderstood concept has received much attention since the first report that 70% of patients (or normals) demonstrate a drop in the intragastric pH < 4 for at least 1 continuous hour in the overnight monitoring period (10 pm to 6 am) despite taking a proton pump inhibitor twice daily. Termed nocturnal gastric acid breakthrough (NAB) occurs most often about 6 to 7 hours after the evening dose of the proton pump inhibitor (PPI), principally between 1 and 4 am on twice-daily PPI. When PPIs are given once daily before breakfast, breakthrough occurs earlier, beginning around 11 pm. This is a class effect, seen in equal frequency with all PPIs, seen with equal frequency in normal, uncomplicated GERD, and Barrett's esophagus (Figures 35-1 and 35-2).

Nocturnal esophageal reflux appears to be extremely rare in normal subjects and patients with uncomplicated GERD. Based on data, nocturnal symptoms occur in less than 15% of patients with erosive esophagitis who are on a PPI once daily, reinforcing the finding on esophageal pH monitoring. However up to 50% of patients with Barrett's esophagus or scleroderma and GERD will have increased overnight esophageal acid exposure during NAB, suggesting it may be important in these patients. This is of particular importance in Barrett's patients as they are often asymptomatic despite nocturnal esophageal acid exposure.

The unifying features of those who will have reflux during NAB are a decreased lower esophageal sphincter pressure and ineffective esophageal motility in the body of the esophagus. In fact, patients with both low sphincter pressure and ineffective motility are

Figure 35-1. Illustrating nocturnal acid breakthrough on twice-daily proton pump inhibitor and resultant gastroesophageal reflux. The bottom tracing shows a drop in intragastric pH to less than 4 overnight, usually seen 6 to 7 hours after the evening dose of proton pump inhibitor. During breakthrough in the upper tracing are 2 reflux episodes (pH drop < 4).

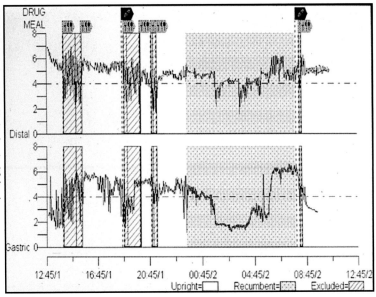

Figure 35-2. pH curves on once-daily proton pump inhibitor demonstrating overnight drop of intragastric pH to less than 4. (Reprinted from Tutuian R, Katz PO, Castell DO. A PPI is a PPI: lessons learned from prolonged intragastric pH monitoring. *Gastroenterology.* 2000;118:A17 [Abstract 332], with permission from Elsevier.)

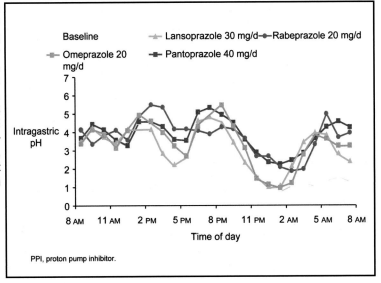

8 times more likely to reflux during gastric acid breakthrough compared to those with normal motility.

The clinical importance and therefore the approach to NAB is the subject of much debate. There are few prospective or controlled clinical studies in which symptoms have been evaluated. Data suggest that 80% to 90% of patients with proven GERD will have adequate nighttime symptom relief on a single daily dose of a PPI. In the patient with continued symptoms, despite twice-daily PPI—and clinical experience suggests frequent symptomatic esophageal acid breakthrough is unusual in most GERD patients—I strongly suggest first reviewing the medication schedule to be certain the PPI is being taken before breakfast and dinner and not before bed as is too often the case. I then perform combined intragastric and intraesophageal reflux monitoring while continuing therapy. If there is nocturnal gastric acid breakthrough and continued reflux, I will consider treatment. It is here that immediate-release omeprazole (IR-OME) sodium bicarbonate (Zegerid) has potential. A randomized, open-label, crossover trial evaluating IR-OME versus delayed-release pantoprazole tablets, both administered to 36 patients with symptomatic nocturnal GERD, reported enhanced control of nocturnal gastric pH with IR-OME at steady state. Immediate-release omeprazole 40 mg and pantoprazole 40 mg were administered once daily (at bedtime or before dinner, respectively) for 6 days and twice daily (before breakfast and at bedtime) on day 7. After 6 days, the median percentage of time that gastric pH was >4 for the nighttime interval (10:00 pm to 6:00 am) was 55% for IR-OME once daily and 26.5% for pantoprazole once daily ($P < .001$). After twice-daily dosing on day 7, the median percentage of time that gastric pH was >4 was 92% and 36.5%, respectively ($P < .001$). A statistically significant difference was also observed when nocturnal pH control rates (i.e., the median percentage of time that gastric pH was >4) for IR-OME 40 mg once daily (day 6) were compared with pantoprazole 40 mg twice daily (day 7) (55% and 34%, respectively; $P < .001$). The median nighttime gastric pH values were 4.7 for IR-OME once daily versus 2.0 and 1.7 for pantoprazole once daily and twice daily, respectively ($P < .001$ for each comparison).

This improved nocturnal pH control suggests that the immediate-release formulation of omeprazole offers a potential advantage in controlling nighttime acidity.

Though no clinical trials have been done and intragastric pH study comparing IR-OME 40 mg suspension, esomeprazole 40 mg, and lansoprazole 30 mg at bedtime (10 pm) showed that IR-OME had the most rapid onset of pH control, specifically controlling intragastric pH better than the comparators in the first 4 hours of the evening when reflux is most likely to occur. I will try to switch to this drug given at bedtime rather than the second PPI dose before dinner in patients who reflux at night on bid PPI. This is my current practice before adding an H_2 receptor antagonist. No studies have been done with the 40-mg capsule, though bioavailability studies suggest the onset of action should be similar to the suspension. My clinical impression is that few GERD patients without Barrett's should require a bedtime PPI because a before-dinner dose was ineffective. Patients with Barrett's esophagus pose a clinical dilemma and are discussed elsewhere.

There appears to be a move on the part of many clinicians as well as managed care organizations in the United States to look to nocturnal H_2 receptor antagonists as less expensive alternatives to increasing proton pump inhibitor dosage in patients with continued nocturnal symptoms on once-daily PPI. Although I cannot refute the logic of this consideration, particularly to save dollar costs of GERD treatment, my clinical experience suggests that this is *not* an optimal approach to patients with on-going frequent symptoms. For the occasional and perhaps predictable nocturnal symptoms, an H_2 blocker might be considered. There are no clinical trials to support the benefit of this approach.

Bibliography

Castell D, Bagin R, Goldlust B, Major J, Hepburn B. Comparison of the effects of immediate-release omeprazole powder for oral suspension and pantoprazole delayed-release tablets on nocturnal acid breakthrough in patients with symptomatic gastro-oesophageal reflux disease. *Aliment Pharmacol Ther.* 2005;21(12):1467-1474.

Katz PO, Anderson C, Khoury R, Castell DO. Gastroesophageal reflux associated with nocturnal gastric acid breakthrough on proton pump inhibitors. *Aliment Pharmacol Ther.* 1998;12:1231-1234.

Katz PO, Ginsberg GG, Hoyle PE, Sostek MB, Monyak JT, Silberg DG. Relationship between intragastric acid control and healing status in the treatment of moderate to severe erosive oesophagitis. *Aliment Pharmacol Ther.* 2007;25(5):617-628.

Peghini PL, Katz PO, Bracy NA, Castell DO. Nocturnal recovery of gastric acid secretion with twice-daily dosing of proton pump inhibitors. *Am J Gastroenterol.* 1998;93:763-767.

What Is the Role of Helicobacter pylori in GERD? Do All Patients With GERD Need to Be Tested for Helicobacter pylori?

Helicobacter pylori is a gram-negative, spiral, flagellated organism that infects the gastric mucosa, leading to chronic gastritis. It has been causally related to duodenal and gastric ulcers, gastric cancer, and gastric mucosa associated lymphoid tissue (MALT) lymphoma. It has been linked to the increased risk for development of ulcer disease in patients on nonsteroidal anti-inflammatory drugs and as a potential contributor to functional or nonulcer dyspepsia.

There are three patterns of infections. Chronic active antral gastritis results in an increase in gastric acid secretion and duodenal ulcer risk. Chronic active corpus gastritis results in a decrease in acid secretion and an increase in gastric ulcer. The bug can result in chronic pangastritis, which is associated with atrophy, gastric intestinal metaplasia, and the perceived and documented increase in gastric cancer.

The relationship of *H. pylori* and gastroesophageal reflux disease has been one of controversy. Some early studies suggested that eradication of *H. pylori* infection in the setting of duodenal ulcer disease would result in an increase in erosive esophagitis and GERD symptoms. Although there are several studies to support this, the weight of the evidence suggests strongly that eradication of *H. pylori* has no effect on the development of heartburn and in fact does not exacerbate GERD symptoms when they are present at baseline. There are also several studies that suggest that in the setting of chronic corpus gastritis and/or panatrophic gastritis, the prevalence of erosive esophagitis, and, in fact,

Figure 36-1. Heartburn after *H. pylori* treatment. Well-done study showing no difference in reflux symptoms 1 and 6 months after *H. pylori* eradication. (Reprinted from Vakil N, Hahn B, McSorley D. Recurrent symptoms and gastro-oesophageal reflux disease in patients with duodenal ulcer treated for Helicobacter pylori infection. *Aliment Pharmacol Ther.* 2000;14(1):45-51, with permission from Blackwell Scientific Publications.)

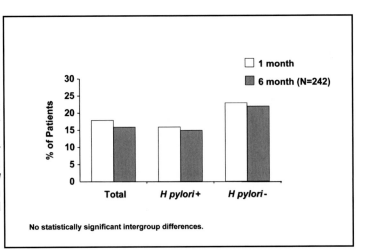

No statistically significant intergroup differences.

the frequency of Barrett's esophagus, is less than in matched groups who do not have infection. This has led to some authorities proposing that *H. pylori* infection might be protective against severe end organ damage in patients with GERD. Frankly, this paradox of *H. pylori* infection being detrimental to the gastric mucosa and at the same time protective of the esophageal mucosa is difficult to reconcile.

When one attempts to work their way through the data, I am comfortable with the following clinical caveats. *H. pylori* infection itself clearly does not cause GERD nor, in fact, have any dramatic effect on symptoms. Eradication of *H. pylori* does not, in my practice, appear to affect the natural history of or the treatment of GERD at all (Figure 36-1). It is, therefore, my recommendation that if the clinical presentation mandates investigation for *Helicobacter* (suspicion of gastric ulcer, duodenal ulcer, or in certain situations functional dyspepsia), testing for *H. pylori* is warranted. In the GERD patient, I find no role in my clinical practice for testing. Should testing be needed, active testing with either a stool antigen test or ureal breath test is preferred to serum immunoglobulin G (IgG) antibody testing as the increased sensitivity and specificity of the former outweigh the upfront cost advantages of the latter. Rapid urease testing of gastric biopsies should be performed if the patient is undergoing endoscopy and testing is indicated. I do not advocate routine biopsy of the gastric mucosa when endoscoping a patient with suspected gastroesophageal reflux disease. If *H. pylori* infection is present for whatever reason, I follow the standard recommendation that the organism be treated and use traditional proton pump inhibitor–based triple therapy for eradication.

The patient seen in the emergency room with noncardiac chest pain is not a candidate for *H. pylori* testing, as the potential etiologies for her pain do not include gastric ulcer and/or duodenal ulcer in my opinion. It is highly unusual in my practice to recall any patient who experienced an improvement in their chronic chest pain with eradication of infection. The question as posed assumes that the noncardiac chest pain is due to reflux, which it may not be. Regardless, there is no reason to suspect that *H. pylori* eradication would make chest pain worse. It is worth commenting that using serology to document infection in this type of patient creates "more trouble than it is worth" as there is no way to determine without a careful history whether or not this represents active or old infection. Ultimately, the best course of action for Ms. Smith would be to evaluate and treat her for noncardiac chest pain with suspected esophageal etiology and not test for *H. pylori* at all.

MS. SMITH WENT TO THE ER WITH CHEST PAIN THAT WAS DETERMINED TO BE NONCARDIAC. SEROLOGIES FOR H. PYLORI WERE FOUND TO BE POSITIVE IN THE ED. I HAVE CONSIDERED TREATING HER BUT HAVE HEARD THAT THIS MAY WORSEN HER REFLUX. WHAT SHOULD I DO?

This question is as much interesting for the decision to do serological testing for *Helicobacter pylori* as the decision to treat the patient or not. A patient seen in the emergency room for noncardiac chest pain is not, in my opinion, a candidate for *Helicobacter* testing, as the potential etiologies for the pain do not include gastric ulcer, duodenal ulcer, or any syndrome that I know to be associated with *H. pylori*. I cannot recall any patient that I have treated who has experienced improvement in their chronic chest pain when *Helicobacter* has been eradicated. As such, this patient should be evaluated for the traditional disease processes associated with noncardiac chest pain, specifically GERD, esophageal motility and sensitivity disorders, chest wall pain, and perhaps chronic gallbladder disease. The latter is a much rarer cause of unexplained chest pain than many think and should be low on the list. A practical approach is to institute an empiric trial of antisecretory therapy, usually twice-daily proton pump inhibitor, for 4 to 8 weeks, make an assessment as to the success of the intervention, and proceed from there. A further

Figure 37-1. Heartburn after *H. pylori* treatment. Well-done study showing no difference in reflux symptoms 1 and 6 months after *H. pylori* eradication. (Reprinted from Vakil N, Hahn B, McSorley D. Recurrent symptoms and gastro-oesophageal reflux disease in patients with duodenal ulcer treated for Helicobacter pylori infection. *Aliment Pharmacol Ther.* 2000;14(1):45-51, with permission from Blackwell Scientific Publications.)

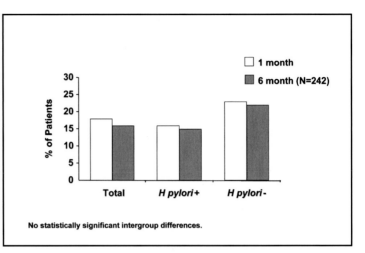

diagnostic work up for GERD, with endoscopy or prolonged reflux monitoring, can be considered and if unrevealing, esophageal function testing can be performed. Nowhere in this "algorithm" is testing for *H. pylori* entertained unless an anatomic abnormality on endoscopy is discovered that is associated with the organism.

It is further worth commenting that using *H. pylori* serology to document infection in this type of patient may create "more trouble than it is worth," as there is no way to determine without a careful history whether or not this represents active or old infection. If testing for *H. pylori* is actually needed, I would recommend testing with either a urea breath test or a stool antigen, both of which have higher sensitivity and specificity than serology and further offer an indication of active infection.

There is little argument that this patient should be treated for *H. pylori*, unless she refuses, due to the background concern that failure to treat will put the patient at risk for gastric cancer. The question as posed, assumes that the noncardiac chest pain is due to reflux, that reflux may worsen, two issues that may not be correct. Regardless, there is no reason to suspect that *H. pylori* eradication would make this chest pain worse, whether it is due to GERD or not (Figure 37-1). Ultimately, the best course of action for Ms. Smith would be to evaluate and treat her for noncardiac chest pain, not test for *H. pylori*, and follow the patient. If as this case outlines, serology is positive, I would treat her without concern of worsening any disease that she has.

CAN MEDICAL THERAPY ALTER THE NATURAL HISTORY OF BARRETT'S ESOPHAGUS?

There are little or no data to suggest that any therapy can alter the natural history of Barrett's, though logic suggests that effect therapy—whether medical or surgical—would do so. Medical therapy has not been systematically studied, nor have the randomized follow-up studies been performed. Studies that have compared medical and surgical therapy for GERD have for the most part excluded patients with Barrett's. Although some observational studies have shown changes in length or squamous overgrowth, showing a real change in the risk for development of dysplasia or cancer has been difficult and in fact cannot be supported with high-level evidence. Although 2 studies support a decrease in dysplasia with proton pump inhibitor (PPI) use compared to no PPI use, methodologic flaws preclude endorsing them enthusiastically. For the most part, these studies are retrospective, do not carefully record antisecretory therapy, and have incomplete follow up. As I have indicated elsewhere, I offer aggressive antireflux therapy to Barrett's patients, being careful to tell them that I cannot "prove" that this will help beyond symptoms. Medical therapy designed to relieve symptoms as the primary end point is perfectly acceptable, although most would use PPIs and not H_2 receptor antagonists. All patients still require surveillance regardless of medical intervention.

The best, most recent data come from a recent single-center study. The authors followed a cohort of patients with different lengths of specialized intestinal metaplasia (SIM), long segments, short segments, and specialized intestinal metaplasia at the squamocolumnar junction. Patients were prospectively followed with a rigorous biopsy protocol with follow up of 44 ± 9.7 months. Patients were on various methods of antisecretory therapy. None of the patients with long-segment Barrett's normalized. All remained with SIM but overall decreased the length of the segment. Development of cancer and dysplasia was the highest in this group. Several of the patients with short segments lost the SIM (30%),

Table 38-1

Multivariate Analysis:
Factors Predictive for Loss of Intestinal Metaplasia

Variable	Odds Ratio (95% CI)	P value
Sex (female)	7.79 (2.4 to 25.5)	0.001*
Race (non-white)	1.28 (0.322 to 5.07)	0.727
Heartburn duration (yr)	1.01 (0.97 to 1.10)	0.040*
Hiatal hernia (number)	2.91 (1.05 to 8.06)	0.737
Barrett's group (EGJSIM+)	6.42 (2.21 to 18.66)	0.001*

CI indicates confidence interval; * indicates statistical significance P < 0.05, + indicates comparison with a measurable segment of SIM (LSBE + SSBE).

Reprinted from Horwhat JD, Baroni D, Maydonovitch C, et al. Normalization of intestinal metaplasia in the esophagus and esophagogastric junction: Incidence and clinical data. *Am J Gastroenterol.* 2007;102(3):497-506.

with overall decrease in length, with a small number developing dysplasia or cancer. In the group with esophagogastric junction SIM, disappearance of the SIM was seen in 67%, none had dysplasia or cancer. Predictors of loss of intestinal metaplasia are outlined in Table 38-1. Although this study does not specifically support a positive effect of therapy, it does suggest that Barrett's metaplasia may regress (or disappear) under surveillance, and perhaps on medical therapy.

Bibliography

Corey KE, Schmitz SM, Shaheen NJ. Does a surgical antireflux procedure decrease the incidence of esophageal adenocarcinoma in Barrett's esophagus? A meta-analysis. *Am J Gastroenterol.* 2003;98(11):2390-2394.

Horwhat JD, Baroni D, Maydonovitch C, et al. Normalization of intestinal metaplasia in the esophagus and esophagogastric junction: Incidence and clinical data. *Am J Gastroenterol.* 2007;102(3):497-506.

Ye W, Chow WH, Lagergren J, et al. Risk of adenocarcinomas of the esophagus and gastric cardia in patients with gastroesophageal reflux diseases and after antireflux surgery. *Gastroenterology.* 2001;121(6):1286-1293.

QUESTION 39

CAN ANTIREFLUX SURGERY ALTER THE NATURAL HISTORY OF BARRETT'S ESOPHAGUS?

Antireflux surgery (fundoplication) has become increasingly popular since the availability and development of laparoscopic approaches have made the procedure more patient friendly. It has been estimated that more than 35,000 laparoscopic Nissen fundoplications are performed annually in the United States. Fundoplication is highly effective in the short-term relief of symptoms, particularly heartburn. Few studies have carefully compared surgery to proton pump inhibitors, particularly long term, nor have critically evaluated long-term symptom relief, quality of life, and prevention of complications. The recent literature sheds light on many of these issues, including development of adenocarcinoma of the esophagus.

Lundell and colleagues recently published 5-year follow-up of a randomized study comparing open fundoplication to medical therapy with omeprazole. Three hundred and forty-four patients were initially treated with omeprazole 20 to 40 mg/day for up to 3 months. Healing of erosive esophagitis and symptom relief was achieved in 310 (76% men), who were subsequently entered into the randomized maintenance trial now with 5- and 7-year follow up.

Patients were randomized to 20 ($n = 139$) or 40 ($n = 16$) mg of omeprazole or to surgery ($n = 155$). The surgical procedure was chosen by the surgeon: Nissen ($n = 100$), (Toupet) ($n = 34$), or a total or posterior partial fundoplication in addition to vagotomy (in patients with concurrent duodenal ulcer) ($n = 10$). Endoscopy was performed at 1, 3, and 5 years after treatment and graded from 0 to 4. Symptoms were assessed: GERD-related, general dyspeptic, and postfundoplication symptoms with a rating from 0 ("no symptoms") to 3 ("severe incapacitating symptoms"). Quality of life was assessed using both the Gastrointestinal Symptoms Rating Scale (GSRS) and Psychological General Well-Being index (PGWB). Some omeprazole failures were treated with either 40 or 60 mg daily, and outcome measures were assessed on this dosage.

The main outcome, treatment failure, was defined as one or more of the following: moderate or severe heartburn or acid regurgitation for 7 or more days before a visit; esophagitis of grade 2 or higher; moderate or severe dysphagia or odynophagia symptoms with mild heartburn or regurgitation more than 3 months after surgery; if allocated to surgery, requirement for omeprazole for more than 8 weeks to control symptoms, or reoperation; if allocated to medical therapy, needing or wanting surgery was considered treatment failure.

Analysis was by intention to treat using life-table analysis. In the surgical group, 14% had symptom relapse, 13% had esophagitis above grade 2, and 5% required more than 8 weeks of omeprazole. For reasons not stated, 11% were otherwise excluded from analysis. In the medical group, 32% had a symptom relapse, 13% had esophagitis above grade 2, and 10% had surgery during the follow-up period. Fewer patients were designated treatment failures in the surgical group than in the group treated with omeprazole 20 mg/day ($P < .001$). When the omeprazole dose was increased to 40 mg/day, statistical significance disappeared. Surgery is thus not a "cure" and does not completely eliminate the need for medical therapy. The study does not specifically address Barrett's but reminds us of relative success of fundoplication compared to medical therapy. Although surgery also reduces Barrett's length in some studies and results in regrowth and overgrowth of squamous tissue, no clear evidence suggests that pateints with Barrett's should have surgery to prevent cancer.

Bibliography

Corey KE, Schmitz SM, Shaheen NJ. Does a surgical antireflux procedure decrease the incidence of esophageal adenocarcinoma in Barrett's esophagus? A meta-analysis. *Am J Gastroenterol.* 2003;98(11):2390-2394.

Horwhat JD, Baroni D, Maydonovitch C, et al. Normalization of intestinal metaplasia in the esophagus and esophagogastric junction: incidence and clinical data. *Am J Gastroenterol.* 2007;102(3):497-506.

Lundell L, Miettinen P, Myrvold HE, et al. Continued (5-year) follow-up of a randomized clinical study comparing antireflux surgery and omeprazole in gastroesophageal reflux disease. *J Am Coll Surg.* 2001;192:172–181.

Ye W, Chow WH, Lagergren J, et al. Risk of adenocarcinomas of the esophagus and gastric cardia in patients with gastroesophageal reflux diseases and after antireflux surgery. *Gastroenterology.* 2001;121(6):1286-1293.

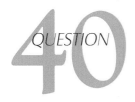

DO EITHER MEDICAL THERAPY OR ANTIREFLUX SURGERY REDUCE THE RISK OF OR PREVENT THE DEVELOPMENT OF ESOPHAGEAL CANCER?

A well-designed case control study by Ye and colleagues provides answers to many important questions regarding reflux disease and adenocarcinoma. The authors reviewed Swedish patient databases from 1965 through 1997 to identify patients hospitalized with GERD-related diagnostic codes; they compared the risk of developing esophageal adenocarcinoma in patients hospitalized with a diagnosis of GERD who were treated with antireflux surgery and in those who did not have operative intervention and hence were, it was assumed, treated medically. A cohort of 35,274 male and 31,691 female patients with a discharge diagnosis of GERD and another cohort of 6406 male and 4671 female patients who underwent antireflux surgery were identified in the Swedish inpatient register. Follow-up was attained through record linkage with several nationwide registers. Standardized incidence ratio (SIR) was used to estimate relative risk of upper gastrointestinal cancers, using the general Swedish population as a reference. Incident cancers were taken into account by excluding cancers that occurred in the first year of follow-up. Because the incidence rates of esophageal cancer were different among men and women, gender was analyzed separately. The authors also examined the incidence of gastric adenocarcinoma as well as squamous cell cancer of the esophagus in this patient cohort.

After excluding the first year's observation, the incidence rate for esophageal adenocarcinoma among males was over six times the risk of the general population (SIR = 6.3; 95% confidence interval [CI] 4.5 to 8.7). Importantly, the relative risk increased as follow-up time increased, rising to an 11-fold increase after 10 or more years of follow-up (P = .03; 95% CI 6.0 to 18.3). All age groups had similar excess risk, with a 2-fold increase seen for gastric cardia adenocarcinoma, but no substantial risk for squamous cell of the esophagus or cancers of the distal stomach. The risk among women was also 6-fold higher (SIR = 6.1; 95% CI 2.9 to 11.2), although women were approximately 15 years older at diagnosis than men (85 versus 71 years). Overall, cancers were 4 times more common in men than women.

The authors point out that for patients with known esophagitis, those who had undergone an endoscopy, who had reflux as their primary admission diagnosis, or who were admitted as emergencies for reflux-related disease had a higher risk of developing esophageal adenocarcinoma.

In contrast to those who did not undergo a surgical procedure, for patients in the antireflux surgery cohort, the relative risk of esophageal cancer did not change materially over time in those followed for 10 or more years. The risk of adenocarcinoma of the gastric cardia was also increased among men operated on for GERD, although there was no increased risk of squamous cell or noncardia stomach cancer.

This study helps to answer many important questions and raises many others. The results strongly support a causal relationship between chronic GERD and the development of adenocarcinoma of the esophagus. Some of the data presented lend support to the assumption that those with what can be characterized as longer-duration and more severe GERD are perhaps at greater risk. Data for those who underwent endoscopy and had a diagnosis of erosive esophagitis, those hospitalized primarily for GERD, and the increase in risk with longevity of follow-up support these contentions. Unfortunately, Barrett's esophagus was not looked for.

The study should also end any debate on the superiority of antireflux surgery to medical therapy. Neither will reliably prevent cancer.

Another recent study, a well-done meta-analysis in which 4678 patient years of follow up in the surgical group and 4906 patient years in the medical group were compared. The incidence of cancer in the surgical group was 3.8 per 1000 patient years compared with 5.3 in the medical group (P = .29), similar to the results of the other case-control study. Ultimately it is fairest to patients to offer the best medical or surgical therapy possible, push hard for regular follow up and surveillance, so that if complications develop they can be managed better if detected early. If therapy—medical or surgical—eliminates Barrett's or delays progression, the patient is better off. I can find no evidence in the literature that either medical or surgical therapy is in and of itself harmful to Barrett's patients. Although smaller surgical series have suggested regression of Barrett's esophagus and even dysplasia, surgery should not be offered as a means of preventing cancer any more than medical therapy. To date, no studies have evaluated endoscopic therapy and their effect on Barrett's esophagus.

Bibliography

Corey KE, Schmitz SM, Shaheen NJ. Does a surgical antireflux procedure decrease the incidence of esophageal adenocarcinoma in Barrett's esophagus? A meta-analysis. *Am J Gastroenterol.* 2003;98(11):2390-2394.

Horwhat JD, Baroni D, Maydonovitch C, et al. Normalization of intestinal metaplasia in the esophagus and esophagogastric junction: incidence and clinical data. *Am J Gastroenterol.* 2007;102(3):497-506.

Ye W, Chow WH, Lagergren J, et al. Risk of adenocarcinomas of the esophagus and gastric cardia in patients with gastroesophageal reflux diseases and after antireflux surgery. *Gastroenterology.* 2001;121(6):1286-1293.

HOW DOES PREGNANCY AFFECT GERD? IS GERD IN PREGNANCY A RISK FOR LONG-TERM REFLUX?

Heartburn is a common symptom that occurs frequently during pregnancy, in any trimester. Although "heartburn" and "gastroesophageal reflux disease (GERD)" have become integrally connected in the medical literature, the 2 terms have distinct connotations. Heartburn is a symptom that is considered highly sensitive and specific for GERD. GERD, on the other hand, is a disorder of abnormal gastroesophageal reflux and its associated complications, of which heartburn is the most common symptom. In the nonpregnant individual, GERD may present with extraesophageal complaints, including cough, hoarseness, vocal changes, and asthma, but the relationship between these symptoms and GERD has not been adequately evaluated in pregnant patients. Because of the close relationship between heartburn and GERD, most studies in this area address pregnancy-related heartburn in the absence of a stringent diagnosis of GERD.

In most women who experience heartburn during pregnancy, the symptoms begin during pregnancy, although less commonly the heartburn may represent a manifestation of underlying GERD. Heartburn may begin in any trimester. In studying pregnant women who experience heartburn, the onset is 52% in the first trimester, 40% in the second trimester, and 8% in the third trimester. The prevalence of heartburn increased with gestational age. Among 607 pregnant women attending an antenatal clinic, 22% experienced heartburn in the first trimester, 39% in the second, and 72% in the third, whereas only 14% of these women reported mild heartburn prior to their pregnancy. Severity also increased throughout pregnancy. Significant predictors of heartburn are increasing gestational age, heartburn before pregnancy, and parity. Maternal age is inversely correlated with heartburn. Race, prepregnancy body mass index, and weight gain in pregnancy do not correlate with the onset of heartburn. Despite its frequent occurrence during pregnancy, heartburn usually resolves after delivery.

Table 41-1

Pathophysiology of GERD During Pregnancy

Potential pathophysiologic mechanisms of heartburn in pregnancy	Contribution
Decreased basal LES pressure	+++
High estrogen + progesterone levels	+++
Loss of intra-abdominal segment of LES	+
Impaired LES contractile response to pharmacologic stimuli	++
Esophageal motility abnormalities	+/−
Increased intra-abdominal pressure	−

In the general population, a number of physiologic abnormalities work in concert to cause GERD, including a defective antireflux barrier, the lower esophageal sphincter (LES); impaired esophageal clearance of the refluxate; an altered mucosal barrier; and abnormalities in gastric function, including delayed gastric emptying. Increased intra-abdominal pressure as a result of the gravid uterus has been proposed as a possible contributing factor to the increased incidence of GERD in pregnancy. However, this alteration does not explain the onset of GERD in the first and early second trimesters, before a change in intra-abdominal pressure is notable. Abnormalities in pregnancy vary with no unifying underlying pathogenetic defect supported in the literature (Table 41-1).

The presentation of GERD in pregnancy does not differ from that of the general population and the diagnosis of GERD during pregnancy is made in much the same fashion as in nonpregnant patients. The cardinal symptom, heartburn, is highly accurate in diagnosing GERD, and in the absence of alarm symptoms such as dysphagia, weight loss, or hematemesis, a presumptive diagnosis of GERD can be made in most patients who develop heartburn during pregnancy. The development of an esophageal stricture during pregnancy has been reported in only a single case report. Regurgitation, characterized by the return of gastric contents into the esophagus or mouth, further supports the diagnosis of GERD when present. Additional diagnostic testing is generally not required for the majority of patients with suspected GERD. Barium radiographs are relatively contraindicated during pregnancy because of their potential for teratogenicity. In the occasional patient who does require testing, upper endoscopy is the test of choice, but should be reserved for patients whose symptoms are refractory to medical therapy or who have suspected complications. Although midazolam is designated as category D and meperidine as category C during pregnancy, the medications are considered generally safe to use in low doses for endoscopy. If possible, however, endoscopy should be delayed until after the first trimester. It is uncommon to require ambulatory pH monitoring during pregnancy, unless the diagnosis of GERD is in doubt.

Bibliography

Diav-Citrin O, Arnon J, Shechtman S, Schaefer C, Van Tonningen MR, Clementi M, DeSantis M, Robert-Gnansia E, Valti E, Malm H, Ornoy A. The safety of proton pump inhibitors in pregnancy: a multicentre prospective controlled study. *Aliment Pharmacol Ther.* 2005;21:269-275.

Katz PO, Castell DO. Gastroesophageal reflux disease during pregnancy. *Gastroenterol Clin N Am.* 1998;27:153-167.

Larson JD. Patatanian E, Miner PB, Rayburn WF, Robinson MG. Double-blind, placebo-controlled study of ranitidine for gastroesophageal reflux symptoms during pregnancy. *Obstet Gynecol.* 1997;90:83-87.

Lewis JH, Weingold AB. The committee on FDA-related matters for the American College of Gastroenterology. The use of gastrointestinal drugs during pregnancy and lactation. *Am J Gastroenterol.* 1985;80:912-923.

Magee LA, Inocencion G, Kamboj L, Rosetti F, Koren G. Safety of first trimester exposure to histamine H_2 blockers: a prospective cohort study. *Digest Dis Sci.* 1996;41:1145-1149.

Marrero JM, Goggin PM, de Caestecker JS, Pearce JM, Maxwell JD. Determinants of pregnancy heartburn. *Br J Obstet Gynaecol.* 1992;99:731-734.

Nikfar S, Abdollahi M, Moretti ME, Magee LA, Koren G. Use of proton pump inhibitors during pregnancy and rates of major malformations: a meta-analysis. *Digest Dis Sci.* 2002;47:1526-1529.

Richter JE. Review article: the management of heartburn in pregnancy. *Aliment Pharmacol Ther.* 2005;22:749-757.

QUESTION 42

WHAT ARE THE TREATMENT OPTIONS FOR GERD IN PREGNANCY?

The safety of medical therapies in the nonpregnant patient is well established. The focus of practitioners who care for pregnant patients with GERD must be the teratogenic potential of antireflux medications (Table 42-1). Concern about teratogenic potential leads many practitioners to avoid pharmacologic agents and pursue conservative care by initially recommending lifestyle modifications, especially for mild symptoms. Chewing gum may also be of benefit for pregnant women with heartburn, as it stimulates salivary bicarbonate production. Other lifestyle and dietary modifications are identical to those in nonpregnant patients, including maintaining a low-fat diet, avoiding alcohol and smoking, and eliminating medications that may exacerbate gastroesophageal reflux (Table 42-2). Pharmacotherapy should ideally be withheld until after the critical period of organogenesis, which ends after the 10th week of gestation.

A summary of medical therapy for GERD in pregnancy is given in Table 42-3.

Antacids should be considered the first line of therapy for symptom relief in pregnant women with heartburn. Antacids, which contain aluminum, magnesium, and calcium, have no Food and Drug Administration (FDA) classification so are generally considered safe for use during pregnancy, although there are limited data regarding fetal safety. However aluminum-containing antacids, especially when taken in high doses, have the potential to cause fetal neurotoxicity. During the last several weeks of pregnancy, magnesium-containing antacids should be avoided because of the tocolytic property of magnesium. Antacids that contain sodium bicarbonate are not considered safe during pregnancy because of the risk for maternal or fetal metabolic alkalosis and fluid overload. Alginic acid (Gaviscon) is usually combined with antacids to cause buffering of gastric acid and works by forming a raftlike barrier to the reflux of gastric contents into the esophagus. It provides adequate relief of heartburn symptoms that develop during pregnancy but has been implicated in adverse fetal outcomes, including fetal distress. Magnesium trisilicate, the compound found in Gaviscon Regular Strength Tablets, can cause fetal nephrolithiasis, hypotonia, respiratory distress, and

Table 42-1
FDA Classification of Drugs During Pregnancy

FDA pregnancy category	Definition
A	Adequate, well-controlled studies in pregnant women have not shown an increased risk of fetal abnormalities.
B	Animal studies have revealed no evidence of harm to the fetus; however, there are no adequate and well-controlled studies in pregnant women, or animal studies have shown an adverse effect, but adequate and well-controlled studies in pregnant women have failed to demonstrate a risk to the fetus.
C	Animal studies have shown an adverse effect and there are no adequate and well-controlled studies in pregnant women, or no animal studies have been conducted and there are no adequate and well-controlled studies in pregnant women.
D	Studies, adequate well-controlled or observational, in pregnant women have demonstrated a risk to the fetus. However, the benefits of therapy may outweigh the potential risk.
X	Studies, adequate well-controlled or observational, in animals or pregnant women have demonstrated positive evidence of fetal abnormalities. The use of the product is **contraindicated** in women who are or may become pregnant.

The Food and Drug Administration. Accessed March 12, 2006. Available at: http://www.fda.gov/fdac/features/2001/301_preg.html. Adapted with permission from the Food and Drug Administration.

cardiovascular impairment when used long-term in high doses. Calcium-based compounds are therefore the preferred first choice of antacids through all trimesters, with magnesium-based compounds (except magnesium trisilicate) a safe option except near the end of pregnancy.

For patients whose symptoms do not respond to antacid therapy, the next option in therapy is H_2-receptor antagonists (H_2RAs). H_2RAs are FDA pregnancy category B, although nizatidine was previously considered a category C drug based on animal studies. Several registries have confirmed in retrospective analyses that exposure to H_2RAs during pregnancy does not appear to increase the rate of major fetal malformations over controls, with rates ranging between 3.1% and 7.4%. There was no increased risk of major fetal malformations (2.1% versus 3.5%) or other adverse gestational outcomes in 178 patients exposed to H_2RAs during pregnancy (88% during the first trimester) when compared with matched controls. Ranitidine is likely needed twice a day to gain a statistically significant improvement in heartburn control versus placebo, with a mean reduction of heartburn intensity of 44.2% versus placebo. Because of weak antiandrogenic properties

Table 42-2

Lifestyle Modifications in GERD

Elevation of head of the bed
Dietary modifications
Low-fat, high-protein diet
Fast for 2 to 3 hours before sleeping
Avoid specific irritants (citrus juices, tomato products, coffee, alcohol)
Avoid chocolate
Stop smoking
Avoid GERD-provocative medications
Anticholinergics
Sedatives/tranquilizers
Theophylline
Prostaglandins
Calcium channel blockers

in cimetidine, there is a theoretical risk of impaired sexual development in male children whose mothers used cimetidine during gestation. There are no reports of this defect occurring in humans. Most of the H_2RA data in human studies are with cimetidine and ranitidine, with limited data on famotidine and nizatidine.

Proton pump inhibitors (PPIs) are the most effective medical therapy currently available to control GERD symptoms and complications. However, their safety in pregnancy is not as well documented as the H_2RAs, and subsequently they should only be used for patients who have severe symptoms that are refractory to other treatments. There are no studies regarding pregnant women with severe GERD complications (Barrett's esophagus, esophageal stricture), but PPI use may also be considered if women are known to harbor one of these conditions prior to gestation. Because animal studies have shown teratogenic effects at large doses, omeprazole is classified as FDA pregnancy category C, but the remainder of the PPIs are category B. A meta-analysis of 5 cohort studies demonstrated a relative risk of 1.18 (95% CI 0.72 to 1.94; P = nonsignificant) for major fetal malformations among 593 PPI-exposed pregnancies. An overall rate of malformations among the exposed pregnancies in this meta-analysis was 2.8%. A recent multicenter prospective cohort study followed 295 pregnancies exposed to omeprazole, 62 to lansoprazole, and 53 to pantoprazole (233, 55, and 47 within the first trimester, respectively). The rates of major congenital abnormalities was 3.6%, 3.9%, and 2.1% respectively, and these rates did not differ from the control group, whose rate of major congenital abnormalities was 3.8%. These studies suggest that PPIs do not necessarily result in a significant increase in major fetal abnormalities. Nonetheless, their use in pregnancy should be approached with caution. When a pregnant woman's symptoms do not respond to antacids, most still

Table 42-3

Summary of Medical Therapy for GERD in Pregnancy

Medication	FDA class	Comments
Antacids Calcium-based Magnesium-based Aluminum-based Alginic acid Magnesium trisilicate Sodium bicarbonate	No FDA classification	Preferred antacid Safe, but has tocolytic properties Possible fetal neurotoxicity May cause fetal distress Fetal toxicity in high doses Not safe due to fluid overload and metabolic acidosis
H$_2$RAs Cimetidine Ranitidine Famotidine Nizatidine	B B B B	
PPIs Omeprazole Lansoprazole Rabeprazole Pantoprazole Esomeprazole	C B B B B	
Others Sucralfate Metoclopramide	B B	Used more commonly for nausea and vomiting of pregnancy

recommend a trial of an H$_2$RA before a PPI, based on the more extensive experience with H$_2$RAs during pregnancy. For women of childbearing age who are taking a PPI prior to pregnancy, it is worthwhile to review the indications for the PPI and the possible teratogenic risks, and reassess the need for chronic therapy prior to any planned pregnancy.

If a woman on chronic antisecretory therapy becomes pregnant during therapy with a PPI, she should be reassured that even though PPI exposure during the first trimester appears to be safe, most would recommend discontinuing the drug at least through the first trimester. Therefore, the need for continued therapy throughout pregnancy should be addressed with the patient as soon as possible so she may make the choice to discontinue the drugs at this critical time.

Promotility agents have played a decreased role in the management of GERD in the nonpregnant patient because potent antisecretory agents have become widely accepted as safe and effective in healing esophagitis and controlling symptoms. Although metoclopramide is categorized as an FDA class B drug and is used in hospitalized patients, it has significant neurologic side effects, including drowsiness, dystonic reactions, and akathisia. Its principal use in pregnancy is for refractory nausea and vomiting of pregnancy. We do not recommend metoclopramide as a treatment for reflux symptoms unless all other options have been exhausted. Tegaserod is an FDA class B drug, but its safety during pregnancy in humans is not well documented. Its use for GERD is not proven so and it cannot currently be recommended for GERD during pregnancy.

Sucralfate is a nonsystemic cytoprotective agent that contains an aluminum salt. As previously discussed, aluminum can cause fetal toxicity, but is likely to be safe during pregnancy because of its poor systemic availability. It is therefore classified as an FDA class B drug. This drug is often recommended in pregnancy based on one study showing improvement in heartburn over placebo.

Most women who develop reflux symptoms during pregnancy experience relief of their symptoms. However, some women, especially those with preexisting GERD, will still require ongoing therapy after delivery during lactation. Certain medications may be transmitted through the breast milk to the nursing infant and the safety of these medications on the newborn is of utmost concern. Antacids, even those containing aluminum, are considered to be safe during lactation. All H_2RAs, and probably all PPIs, are excreted in breast milk. H_2RAs are considered to be safe; however, one animal study suggested that nizatidine caused growth retardation in nursing pups. Nizatidine is therefore the only H_2RA not recommended for use by lactating mothers. The concentration of PPIs in breast milk and the safety of PPIs on the nursing infant have not been adequately investigated. PPIs are also not recommended for use during lactation. Those women who require continued GERD therapy postpartum should avoid PPIs during lactation or discontinue nursing.

All pregnant patients should be carefully counseled so they can make informed choices on how to be treated, if at all, during pregnancy.

Bibliography

Diav-Citrin O, Arnon J, Shechtman S, Schaefer C, Van Tonningen MR, Clementi M, DeSantis M, Robert-Gnansia E, Valti E, Malm H, Ornoy A. The safety of proton pump inhibitors in pregnancy: a multicentre prospective controlled study. *Aliment Pharmacol Ther.* 2005;21:269-275.

Katz PO, Castell DO. Gastroesophageal reflux disease during pregnancy. *Gastroenterol Clin N Am.* 1998;27: 153-167.

Larson JD. Patatanian E, Miner PB, Rayburn WF, Robinson MG. Double-blind, placebo-controlled study of ranitidine for gastroesophageal reflux symptoms during pregnancy. *Obstet Gynecol.* 1997;90:83-87.

Lewis JH, Weingold AB. The committee on FDA-related matters for the American College of Gastroenterology. The use of gastrointestinal drugs during pregnancy and lactation. *Am J Gastroenterol.* 1985;80:912-923.

Magee LA, Inocencion G, Kamboj L, Rosetti F, Koren G. Safety of first trimester exposure to histamine H_2 blockers: a prospective cohort study. *Digest Dis Sci.* 1996;41:1145-1149.

Marrero JM, Goggin PM, de Caestecker JS, Pearce JM, Maxwell JD. Determinants of pregnancy heartburn. *Br J Obstet Gynaecol.* 1992;99:731-734.

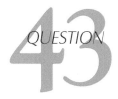

A 45-Year-Old Gentleman Comes to You Following a Laparoscopic Nissen Fundoplication 5 Years Ago. He Now Has Recurrent GERD Symptoms. How Common Is This?

The decision to send a patient to surgery for GERD is not straightforward. If the patient is intolerant of or allergic to proton pump inhibitors (PPIs), the decision is relatively easy for me. In patients who are on high doses of PPI, those with reflux-related lung disease, those who cannot or choose not to afford PPIs, and those with regurgitation due to non-acid reflux surgery, the alternative is often considered. In making this decision, the patient must weigh the risks and benefits of surgery versus long-term medical therapy and consider the possibility of relapse even if surgery is initially successful.

There have been 3 well-done published randomized trials comparing available medical to surgery therapy for GERD. The earliest showed superiority of open antireflux surgery compared to lifestyle modification and antacids, the next trial showed short-term superiority of antireflux surgery (open fundoplication) to histamine receptor antagonist with or without metoclopramide. Each of these trials was "criticized" because at the time of publication, medical therapy had advanced to the point that the standard of practice had progressed to more potent antisecretory therapy. When the patients in the former trial were followed up 10 to 13 years after randomization, a high return to medical therapy (60%) was seen after antireflux surgery, though return of reflux was not specifically sought. The third, a well-designed, multicenter randomized trial published 5-year follow up of 310 patients randomized to open fundoplication or omeprazole 20 mg/day

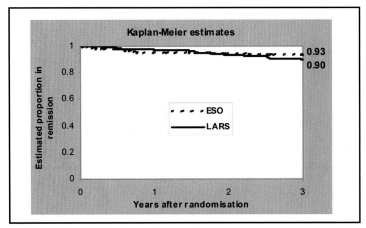

Figure 43-1. Three-year outcomes for laparoscopic antireflux surgery (LARS) versus medical (esomeprazole, ESO) therapy.

(increasing as needed to 60 mg/day) in 2001. There was a small but not statistically significant advantage for surgery, which continued at the 7-year follow up. Fundoplication technique was not standardized and was performed open, whereas today's standard is laparoscopic.

Three recent studies offer more insight into this comparison. All are abstracts, so some details are missing that temper any definite conclusion. All compared medical and surgical therapy directly. The first is a new randomized trial, the other two are long-term follow up of the third study above.

The 3-year results of an ongoing open, parallel group, multicenter, randomized, controlled trial conducted in 11 European countries compares laparoscopic antireflux surgery to medical therapy. Laparoscopic antireflux surgery (LARS) was completed according to a standardized protocol, always compromising a total fundoplication and a posterior crural repair. Medical treatment was with esomeprazole 20 mg once daily, which could be increased stepwise to 20 mg twice daily in cases of incomplete GERD control. The primary outcome variable was time to treatment failure assessed by life-table analysis. Treatment failure was defined as insufficient control of GERD. In the medical group, it was the need for therapy beyond esomeprazole 40 mg/day and in the LARS group, the need for medical therapy (exclusive of antacids) or an additional operation.

A total of 554 patients were randomized (esomeprazole: n = 266; LARS: n = 288). Baseline demographics and disease characteristics were similar between study arms. The estimated proportion of patients who remained in remission was 93% for ESO and 90% for LARS (Figure 43-1).

Over the first 3 years of this long-term study, both continuous esomeprazole treatment and laparoscopic total fundoplication were effective and well-tolerated therapeutic strategies for control of GERD.

The 12-year follow up results of the first randomized study of safety and efficacy comparing omeprazole with open antireflux therapy has been reported in preliminary form. This was originally designed as an open, randomized, multicenter study. Chronic GERD patients with esophagitis (N = 310) and who were considered candidates for surgery

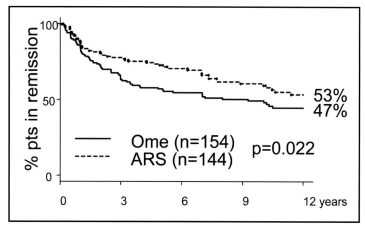

Figure 43-2. Long-term outcomes in patients treated for reflux. ARS = antireflux surgery; OME = omeprazole.

were randomized to either maintenance treatment with omeprazole or open fundoplication. The primary variable was time to treatment failure (recurrence of at least moderate heartburn or recurrence of esophagitis or need for other therapy on the initial dose of omeprazole). The profile and severity of postfundoplication complaints, as well as tolerability of drug were also reported.

The estimated proportions of patients in sustained remission after 12 years were 53% and 47% in the antireflux surgery (ARS) and omeprazole groups, respectively ($P = .022$) (Figure 43-2). During the study, 38% of ARS patients required maintenance proton pump inhibitor (PPI) treatment and 15% of omeprazole patients were operated on. Seven patients in the ARS group were reoperated on. The average dose in the omeprazole group after 1 and 10 years was 24 and 26 mg, respectively. Compared with the omeprazole group, more patients in the ARS group complained of dysphagia, inability to belch and vomit, and rectal flatulence. The prevalence of these symptoms remained similar over time. Both therapies were otherwise well tolerated.

The authors conclude that both long-term PPI therapy and fundoplication are safe and effective strategies for treatment of chronic GERD. Surgery was superior to omeprazole for keeping patients in sustained remission over the observation period, but proportionally more in the surgical group needed additional treatment. Postfundoplication complaints remain a problem. No major side effects were reported in the medical arm. The striking part of these results are the very high relapse rates in both arms and are quite divergent from our clinical impression of long term "success" of medical therapy. The results differ from a long-term observational study showing greater than 90% sustained endoscopic and clinical remission on omeprazole with similar mean and median doses as in this study.

This preliminary report lacks detail on the frequency of follow up, how many patients had endoscopic relapse, what compliance was with therapy, etc. Nevertheless, these are a sizable number of patients followed for over a decade with a clear message. Surgery offers excellent short-term success. Although many will remain successfully treated, a substantial minority will relapse and require additional treatment. Side effects from surgery should not be trivialized.

Overall, informed consent should include careful explanation of both short- and long-term outcomes as well as side effects for both methods of treatment. Medical therapy may not be as "good as advertised." We must carefully follow patients to assure optimal results and be prepared to make adjustments in PPI dose as needed for optimal outcomes. Careful attention to new information on long-term side effects of PPIs is mandatory as most patients will choose medical therapy.

Bibliography

Behar J, Sheahan DG, Biancani P, et al. Medical and surgical management of reflux esophagitis. A 38-month report of a prospective clinical trial. *N Engl J Med.* 1975;293(6):263-268.

Lundell L, Hatlebakk JG, Attwood S, et al. The Lotus trial—comparing esomeprazole to laparascopic anti-reflux surgery for the management of chronic gastroesophageal reflux disease: a 3-year interim analysis. *Gastroenterology.* 2007;132(4):A107 [Abstract 753].

Lundell L, Miettinen P, Myrvold HE, et al. Continued (5-year) follow up of a randomized clinical study comparing antireflux surgery and omeprazole in gastroesophageal reflux disease. *J Am Coll Surg.* 2001;192(2):172-179.

Lundell L, Miettinen P, Myrvold H, et al. Anti-reflux surgery compared with maintenance omeprazole for reflux esophagitis. Results after 12 years. *Gastroenterology.* 2007;132(4):A107 [Abstract 754].

Spechler SJ. Comparison of medical and surgical therapy for complicated gastroesophageal reflux disease in veterans. The Department of Veterans Affairs Gastroesophageal Reflux Disease Study Group. *N Engl J Med.* 1992; 326(12):786-792.

WHAT IS THE ASSOCIATION OF OBESITY AND GERD?

The prevalence of obesity (defined as body mass index [BMI] > 30) has increased from approximately 15% in 1980 (National Health and Nutrition Examination Survey II [NHANES II]) to almost 31% (NHANES Continuous 1999 to 2000). Standard textbooks and articles refer to weight reduction as an important component of treatment. The literature is replete with reports attempting to substantiate or refute the long-held assumption of the association between obesity and GERD. Obesity may be a risk factor for the development of Barrett's esophagus and adenocarcinoma of the esophagus. Controversies abound in this area.

The most important pathophysiologic abnormality in GERD is a decrease in lower esophageal sphincter (LES) pressure, often in association with a transient lower esophageal sphincter relaxation (TLESR). The resting LES pressure in normal controls is decreased by fat, which also increases the frequency of TLESRs, thus predisposing to symptoms of GERD. It should be noted, however, that TLESR frequency may be increased by gastric fundal distension, so any meal, regardless of its composition, will to some degree promote reflux. Further, the speed at which one eats will affect the frequency of postprandial reflux. Meals eaten quickly (less than 5 minutes) will produce more postprandial reflux than meals eaten slowly (over 30 minutes).

Basal LES pressure in the morbidly obese appears to be similar to those of ideal body weight, whereas an increase in the presence of a hiatal hernia in patients with obesity and GERD has been described. In more recent studies, however, the pressure morphology within and across the gastroesophageal junction has been shown to be altered with obesity in a fashion that would augment the flow of gastric juice into the esophagus. The increase in intra-abdominal pressure in obese patients may also cause the cephalad movement of a hiatus hernia and thus predisposing them to reflux. Gastric volume has been shown to be normal as has gastric emptying in the obese patient. Gastric acid production is also likely normal, though one study did show a higher maximal gastric acid response to gastrin stimulation. A recent study provided preliminary evidence for the presence of an association between obesity and intraesophageal acid exposure and this association seemed to be mostly mediated by waist circumference as well. An increase in acid sensitivity in obese subjects was seen in one study compared to those of normal body weight. Putting all these various studies together, obese patients are more likely to have a hiatal hernia, increased intragastric pressure, and an augmented gastroesophageal pressure gradient, providing the ideal situation for reflux to occur. There are data supporting the role of abdominal obesity, reflected as a greater waist circumference, as a mediator of the effect of obesity on gastric pressure. In addition, gastric emptying is delayed after a large meal and in meals of high caloric density so that a large meal containing a high degree of fat would perhaps predispose to TLESRs and a greater risk for reflux.

There is controversy related to symptomatic GERD and its relationship to obesity. A population-based study did not reveal any relationship between BMI and GERD symptoms. A meta-analysis suggested an association between BMI and the presence of GERD in the United States. Other large studies have shown that GERD is common among the overweight. In a cross-sectional study, a positive association between BMI and GERD symptoms was found in women. An increase in BMI of more than 3.5, as compared with no weight changes, was associated with an increased risk of frequency of GERD symptoms. A BMI greater than 30 kg per m^2 was associated with almost 3 times higher risk of frequent reflux symptoms. Weight gain has been associated with an increased risk of symptoms of GERD and weight loss associated with a decrease in risk. A recent meta-analysis also demonstrated a dose-response relationship between BMI and the risk of reporting symptoms of GERD among both men and women. In the same meta-analysis, both overweight (BMI 25 to 29) and obesity (BMI > 30) were associated with an increased risk for GERD symptoms, with odds ratios of 1.43 and 1.94, respectively ($P < .001$). It has also been suggested that an increasing BMI is associated with an incremental increase in the risk of developing GERD symptoms. When severity of symptoms is examined, the difference is not as dramatic. Studies have shown contradictory results when assessing esophageal acid exposure in obesity. One study found that 64% of patients in a bariatric surgery program had abnormal ambulatory 24-hour esophageal acid exposure compared to only 30% asymptomatic volunteers ($P = .04$), though the sample numbers were small. In addition, heartburn, acid regurgitation, dysphagia, and asthma were more prevalent in the bariatric surgery patients than in the general population. A second study of 50 consecutive obese patients referred for bariatric surgery found no difference than the general population on 24-hour ambulatory pH-metry and endoscopy. An association between increasing abdominal girth has been seen but not consistent in blacks or Asians. Overall, however, the weight of the epidemiologic evidence would seem to support a connection or an association between gastroesophageal reflux disease and obesity.

Epidemiological studies looked at have the association of obesity and mucosal abnormalities. Obesity increases the risk for GERD symptoms, erosive esophagitis, and esophageal adenocarcinoma. The risk seems to progressively increase with increasing weight. Even controlling for a hiatus hernia, BMI is a risk factor for erosive esophagitis. Obesity is an independent risk factor for the development of Los Angeles grades C and D erosive esophagitis but not the milder grades, although the statistical evidence suggesting a relationship was weak. Similar results are seen in the Chinese. Patients were studied for risk factors associated with GERD. Logistic regression analysis identified several independent risk factors for erosive esophagitis including BMI. The odds for higher degrees of erosive esophagitis were higher as BMI rose. Though some studies do not show an increase in erosive esophagitis in obese patients with GERD, the balance of the evidence seems to favor a relationship.

It is of greatest concern that there has been a well-documented association between BMI and carcinoma of the esophagus and gastric cardia. These are perhaps the most concerning and distressing links between obesity and its effect on the natural history and severity of gastroesophageal reflux disease.

IS BARIATRIC SURGERY GOOD FOR REFLUX?

Nonsurgical weight loss usually results in no effect on symptoms, endoscopic findings, or pH monitoring. However, a recent study showed a reduction of nearly 40% in the risk of frequent GERD symptoms among women with a decrease in BMI of more than 3.5 as compared with women without a change in body mass index (BMI) (odds ratio 0.64). Another study of 34 patients with a BMI greater than 23 found that GERD symptoms improved by 75% from baseline with weight loss (Figure 45-1). A direct correlation between weight loss and symptom score was seen. The beneficial effect of weight reduction in improvement of reflux symptoms has been suggested after bariatric procedures as well. In these studies, however, the independent effect of weight loss on reflux symptoms is hampered as the procedure has an antireflux component. There is a near-complete cessation of acid production in a small proximal gastric pouch and complete diversion of duodenal contents, making the Roux-en-Y gastric bypass in theory the optimal antireflux procedure. There are unfortunately no prospective studies examining the relationship of obesity and the outcome of traditional medical therapy in GERD nor if obesity affects pharmacodynamics or pharmacokinetics of proton pump inhibitors.

I approach obese patients with GERD in a similar fashion to those with reflux disease who are of ideal body weight as there are no definitive studies that address outcomes of traditional medical therapy in this subset of patients. In considering alternatives to medical therapy, the available, approved endoscopic therapies (endoluminal gastric plication, radiofrequency energy ablation) have not been directly studied in those with BMI greater than 30 or 35 kg/m^2. Antireflux surgery is always an option in patients with gastroesophageal reflux disease, with a symptomatic response to proton pump inhibitors. Current data suggest that both fundoplication and Roux-en-Y gastric bypass are effective in long-term treatment of GERD. Fundoplication has lower perioperative risks and excellent outcomes in overweight patients (BMI 25 to 29.9) with GERD without obesity-related morbidity. Patients with class II (BMI 35 to 39.9) with weight-related comorbidities or class III (BMI > 40) irrespective of other comorbidities should probably be offered a bariatric

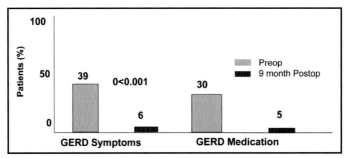

Figure 45-1. Observational, nonrandomized study ($N = 606$) showing effect of weight loss on GERD symptoms. (Reprinted from Nelson LG, Gonzalez R, Haines K, Gallagher SF, Murr MM. Amelioration of gastroesophageal reflux symptoms following Roux-en-Y gastric bypass for clinically significant obesity. *Am Surg.* 2005;71[11]:950-953, with permission from Southeastern Surgical Congress.)

Table 45-1

Suggested Pathophysiologic Factors Predisposing Obese Patients to GERD

Mechanical	Increased intragastric pressure and augmented GEPG Increased incidence of hiatal hernia Increased sensitivity of esophagus to acid exposure
Physiological	Increased bile and pepsin composition of gastric content and increased outputs of bile and pancreatic secretions Higher maximal gastric acid response to graded intravenous pentagastrin Lack of suppression of basal gastric acid secretion after intravenous secretin Increased incidence of Helicobacter pylori Reduced cholecystokinin-stimulated pancreatic enzyme secretion, bile acid emptying, and gastrin release

procedure. A variety of bariatric procedures have been reported to reduce acid reflux and symptoms. There are a multitude of studies looking at the outcome measures of antireflux surgeries based on BMI. One study found a high rate of recurrence (31%) in patients with BMI greater than 30 kg/m^2, compared to a recurrence rate of 8% in patients with BMI between 25 and 29.9 and only 4.5% in patients with BMIs less than 25 kg/m^2. Another found no difference in symptom scores after antireflux surgery in those of normal body weight compared to those obese. In a multivariate analysis of factors predicting symptomatic outcomes after laparoscopic antireflux procedures, obesity was not found to be associated with worse outcomes. Similarly, in a review of 505 patients having undergone laparoscopic antireflux procedures grouped by BMI, no association was found between

Table 45-2
Weight Loss: GERD and Complications

• Recommended for patients with GERD
• Results inconsistent
• Uncontrolled studies suggest improvement in GERD symptoms
• No data on weight loss and esophageal adenocarcinoma

BMI and complications or anatomic failure. In general, these patients present a difficult problem for the surgeons and we await the systematic study of bariatric surgery on its effect on gastroesophageal reflux disease.

Although the balance of the epidemiologic data support a relationship between obesity and GERD, as logic would suggest, true cause and effect cannot be documented. Obese patients do have the right environment for reflux to occur (Table 45-1). Unfortunately, it is difficult to predict what degree of weight loss is required to alter the pressure profile across the gastroesophageal junction and improve other mechanical factors. Achieving and maintaining ideal body weight has a variety of beneficial heath effects and this should supersede GERD as the primary impetus to lose weight (Table 45-2).

IS THERE A GENDER DIFFERENCE IN REFLUX DISEASE? DOES THIS AFFECT TREATMENT?

Despite the prevalence of and large body of research in the field of gastroesophageal reflux, surprisingly, there are scant data addressing the features of GERD in women distinct from men. The clinical impression from personal observations and few studies suggest that the common presentations of GERD are similar in men as in women. In a recent study attempting to examine the features of GERD in women, a similar percentage experienced heartburn, regurgitation, dysphagia, noncardiac chest pain, cough, and/or wheezing as men in the study. There was a trend to a higher frequency of symptoms and slightly increased severity of symptoms in women compared to men; however, the clinical importance of this difference is unclear. The prevalence of hiatal hernia was similar in men and women as well. Though not seen in this study, there does, however, appear to be a difference in the esophageal findings on endoscopy. Patients with erosive esophagitis are more likely to be men, women more likely to have nonerosive disease (heartburn and a normal endoscopy). Some have suggested that this is the result of different symptom sensitivity and/or to different patterns of health-seeking behavior between the sexes; however, neither has been documented. In the aforementioned study, twice as many men had Barrett's (23%) compared to women (14%), $P < .05$. At this time the gender ratio for esophageal adenocarcinomas is 8:1 male to female. Again, the reasons for this dramatic difference in this complication is at present unknown. Exposure to acid reflux may be slightly higher in normal or symptomatic men; however, this does not appear of clinical importance. There is no current evidence that women respond any differently to antisecretory therapy or antireflux surgery than men The only change in treatment based on gender should be in the pregnant patient.

This relationship between GERD and obesity was assessed directly using a questionnaire assessing the severity, duration, and frequency of GERD symptoms in participants from the Nurses Health Study. The authors examined the association between body mass index (BMI) and GERD symptoms in these women. Twenty-two percent had symptoms at least weekly, with 55% describing their symptoms as moderate in severity. Women with a BMI greater than 22.5 had an increased odds ratio for frequent symptoms, which increased to an odds ratio of almost three for those with a BMI greater than 35. Of perhaps greater importance, even in women with a normal BMI at baseline, weight gain resulting in an increase of more than 3.5 in BMI increased odds of frequent reflux symptoms compared to those with stable weight. It appears from this study that weight gain of any type is associated with an increase in reflux symptoms. Men were not studied so the differences in gender cannot be ascertained.

In summary, GERD is common in women, likely as frequent as men. Women may have more frequent and severe symptoms but have a lower incidence of Barrett's esophagus and, to date, esophageal adenocarcinoma. Regardless of the differences, management principles are similar to men and outcomes excellent with proper therapy. Despite the lower incidence of Barrett's esophagus, women should still discuss the need (option) for screening for this condition with their care provider. There is a clear relationship between BMI and reflux symptoms in women, unstudied in men. GERD symptoms are common in pregnancy but can be safely and successfully managed.

Bibliography

Jacobson BC, Somers SC, Fuchs CS, et al. Body mass index and symptoms of gastroesophageal reflux in women. *N Engl J Med.* 2006;354(22):2340-2348.

Lin M, Gerson LB, Lascar R, et al. Features of gastroesophageal reflux disease in women. *Am J Gastroenterol.* 2004;99:1442-1447.

Locke GR, Talley NJ, Gett SL, et al. Prevalence and clinical spectrum of gastroesophageal reflux: a population based study in Olmsted County, Minnesota. *Gastroenterology.* 1997;112:1448-1456.

Nilsson M, Johnsen R, Ye W, et al. Prevalence of gastro-oesophageal reflux symptoms and the influence of age and sex. *Scand J Gastroenterol.* 2004;39:1040-1045.

Ter RB, Johnston BT, Castell DO. Influence of age and gender on gastroesophageal reflux in symptomatic patients. *Dis Esophagus.* 1998;11(2):106-108.

What Are the Ethnic Differences in GERD Presentations?

The difference in GERD in various ethnic groups is understudied. If one looks at the prevalence of heartburn in the U.S. population and attempts to divide it by race, the data are conflicting. If one looks at erosive esophagitis as an end point, GERD appears to be more common in white men than non-white men. Heartburn on the other hand, appears to be similar across ethnic groups. A study of the prevalence of weekly GERD symptoms among various ethnic groups in the Houston area found no statistical difference between whites, blacks, Asians, Hispanics, Native Americans, and other ethnic groups (Figure 47-1). This may not be the same when other countries are surveyed, but appears to be representative of the U.S. population. Erosive esophagitis appears to be more common in Caucasians than in African Americans, though the reason for this is undefined. Although clearly understudied, Barrett's esophagus continues to be more prevalent among Caucasians than Hispanics, Native Americans, and African Americans. On the other hand, if the ethnic backgrounds are looked at percentage wise, the prevalence of Barrett's is similar in Caucasians and Hispanics, with an overall background prevalence of 3% to 6%. Patients of Asian descent also have a similar prevalence of GERD symptoms and currently have a decreased incidence of erosive esophagitis and/or Barrett's esophagus.

Ultimately, the following comments are reflective of the literature and what I see in practice. Heartburn does not appear to discriminate by race or ethnic background. The end organ complications of GERD, erosive esophagitis, Barrett's esophagus, and likely esophageal adenocarcinoma, are more common in Caucasians. None of these differences affect my clinical management or approach to the patient, though one might argue that the threshold for endoscopic screening for Barrett's esophagus be different in African Americans and Asians, those at lower risk for the development of complications. As I am a "Barrett's screener," I offer screening endoscopy to all patients whom I see with chronic GERD, regardless of ethnic background.

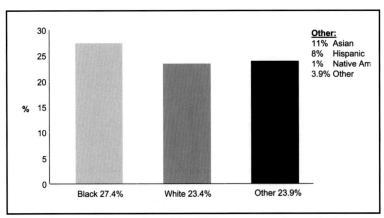

Figure 47-1. Prevalence of weekly GERD among various ethnic groups (VA hospital, Houston). (Reprinted from El-Serag HB, Petersen NJ, Carter J, et al. Gastroesophageal reflux among different racial groups in the United States. *Gastroenterology.* 2004;126[7]:1692-1699, with permission from Elsevier.)

Bibliography

Chiocca JC, Almos JA, Salis GB, et al. Prevalence, clinical spectrum and atypical symptoms of gastro-oesophageal reflux in Argentina: a nationwide population-based study. *Aliment Pharmacol Ther.* 2005;22(4):331-342.

Diaz-Rubio M, Moren-Elola-Olaso C, Rey E, et al. Symptoms of gastro-oesophageal reflux: prevalence, severity, duration, and associated factors in a Spanish population. *Aliment Pharmacol Ther.* 2004;19(1):95-105.

El-Serag HB, Petersen NJ, Carter J, et al. Gastroesophageal reflux among different racial groups in the United States. *Gastroenterology.* 2004;126(7):1692-1699.

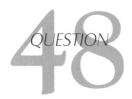

WHICH PATIENTS WITH BARRETT'S SHOULD BE REFERRED FOR PHOTODYNAMIC THERAPY?

The use of ablative therapy for Barrett's esophagus is an area of long-term debate in the gastrointestinal (GI) literature. As one answers this question, it is important to keep in mind that the goals of therapy for Barrett's esophagus might best be placed into the following:

1. Reduce mortality.
2. Reduce cancer.
3. Improve the quality of life.

The latter most simply and straightforwardly can be improved by appropriately treating symptoms of reflux and developing rapport with the patient. A clear understanding of the long-term outcomes, including the risk for cancer, is crucial in managing these patients. Ultimately, the average patient with Barrett's esophagus is unclear as to the ultimate risk of cancer and/or mortality in this disease. A recent study suggested that patients' perception of their risk of developing cancer ranges from 1 in 10 to 1 in 1000. Although ultimately screening and surveillance for the development of dysplasia are paramount, the consideration of active therapy for eliminating Barrett's tissue has been discussed and attempted. As mentioned in other parts of the book, there is little evidence that proton pump inhibitor (PPI) therapy alone can eliminate Barrett's mucosa, though in observational studies, PPIs have been shown to reduce the risk of dysplasia and perhaps be associated with regression or disappearance of short segments.

Ablative technologies are myriad and include laser, argon plasma coagulation, multipolar electrocoagulation (biCap therapy), cryotherapy, and photodynamic therapy (PDT). The most recent ablative technology to enter the field is radiofrequency ablation using what has been named the Halo system.

Each of the ablative technologies has met with their proponents and detractors, specifically multipolar electrocoagulation and argon plasma coagulation. These two

Figure 48-1. Methods to "eliminate" Barrett's.

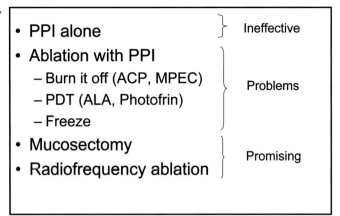

- PPI alone ⎫ Ineffective
- Ablation with PPI ⎫
  - Burn it off (ACP, MPEC) ⎬ Problems
  - PDT (ALA, Photofrin)
  - Freeze ⎭
- Mucosectomy ⎫ Promising
- Radiofrequency ablation ⎭

technologies have been shown to result in "complete ablation of Barrett's" in a range of 0% to 100% of patients treated. Adverse events include transient chest pain, stricture formation, and unfortunately anecdotal reports of perforation. Perhaps the most critical issue is the finding that there are "buried Barrett's glands" beneath the neosquamous mucosa complicating surveillance and suggesting that neither of these technologies provides reliable ablation. PDT, which uses various frequencies of ultraviolet light to ablate tissue, has been studied for many years and is the most carefully studied ablative technology to date. Several trials have shown the ability to ablate Barrett's tissue and decrease and/or ablate high-grade dysplasia and intramucosal cancer in various frequencies. The technology is limited by its complications, which include stricture in somewhere between 10% and 35%, the development of atrial fibrillation, pleural effusions, and photosensitivity. The well-publicized randomized controlled trial of PDT plus PPI therapy twice daily versus proton pump inhibitor therapy alone for patients with Barrett's and high-grade dysplasia has demonstrated superior control of high-grade dysplasia and a decreased development in cancer in up to 3 years of reported follow up compared to PPIs alone. This study, however, does not eliminate cancer (13% in the high-grade group still develop cancer compared to 37% in the PPI group) and did not completely ablate the high-grade dysplasia (77% versus 39% in the PPI group). As such, PDT does not eliminate the lesion nor prevent cancer. Nevertheless, it has remained a viable option for patients with high-grade dysplasia who do not wish to have, or are poor candidates for, surgical intervention.

The Halo 360 ablation catheter uses high-power rapid delivery radiofrequency energy via multiple electrodes to circumferentially ablate Barrett's tissue. Clinical trials are in progress for low-grade dysplasia, high-grade dysplasia, and Barrett's esophagus with no dysplasia, with early reports being quite promising. Complete ablation of intestinal metaplasia has been seen in 70% to 90%, no strictures, no perforations, and at present no buried glands. This promising technology awaits further publication and observation.

The final area of discussion, subject to minimal debate today, is whether nondysplastic Barrett's should be ablated. Simply stated, the answer is likely no, as current data suggest that the natural history of the disease (rate of development of dysplasia or cancer) is unaffected when nondysplastic or, in fact, low-grade dysplasia is ablated. Therefore at the time of this writing, I cannot recommend ablation for anything other than high-grade dysplasia and this should only be done after carefully explaining all options to the patient.

Therapies for Barrett's esophagus are summarized in Figure 48-1.

Bibliography

Ell C, May A, Pech O, et al. Curative endoscopic resection of early esophageal adenocarcinomas (Barrett's cancer). *Gastrointest Endosc.* 2007;65(1):3-10.

Overholt BF, Lightdale CJ, Wang KK, et al. Photodynamic therapy with porfimer sodium for ablation of high-grade dysplasia in Barrett's esophagus: international, partially blinded, randomized phase III trial. *Gastrointest Endosc.* 2005;62(4):488-498.

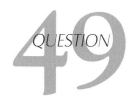
I Know That Reflux and Eosinophilic Esophagitis Can Lead to Dysphagia and Eosinophils on Esophageal Biopsy. How Do I Differentiate These Two Diseases?

Eosinophilic esophagitis is a disease process seen more frequently in adults over the past 5 to 10 years. In its classic presentation, it is seen in young men with recurrent intermittent solid food dysphagia and a history of food impaction. As the disease is discovered in increased frequency, the diagnosis is being entertained and made in adults of any age, gender, and ethnic background with unexplained dysphagia, chest pain, and refractory reflux symptoms. It is in the latter 2 clinical situations that the differentiation between reflux disease and eosinophilic esophagitis becomes a clinical challenge.

As defined, eosinophilic esophagitis is a disease of unknown etiology characterized by eosinophilic inflammation of the esophageal mucosa, classically defined as greater than 15 to 25 eosinophils per high power field in the absence of known causes of eosinophilia. The disease is limited to the esophagus, though a small minority will have peripheral eosinophilia. Gastroesophageal reflux disease results in esophageal mucosal inflammation, which may include eosinophils but almost always at lower than 5 per high power field. The classic reflux lesion is characterized by papillary elongation, intraepithelial neutrophils, and eosinophils. The histologic changes are usually found in the distal esophagus, which is the most common area biopsied. Eosinophilic esophagitis, in contrast, is characterized by a paucity of other inflammatory cells, the intense eosinophilic infiltration that is patchy but is seen in both the proximal and the distal esophagus. On endoscopic evaluation, the diseases are differentiated by their mucosal findings, with

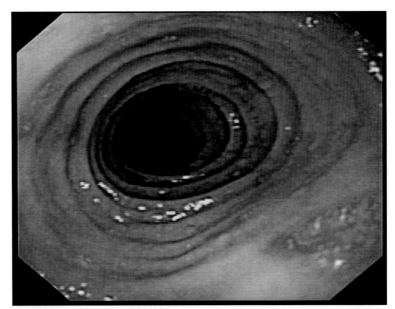

Figure 49-1. Endoscopic appearance of eosinophilic esophagitis illustrating multiple concentric rings and serosal (white) eosinophalic "absesses."

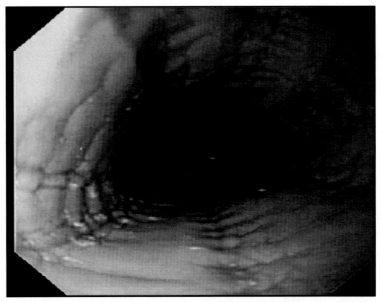

Figure 49-2. Endoscopic appearance of eosinophilic esophagitis. Demonstrates linear furrows or corrugations with subtle ring formation.

eosinophilic esophagitis characterized by mucosal rings, linear furrows in the esophageal lumen, multiple white papules and plaques, or nodules that classically have eosinophilic infiltration (Figures 49-1 and 49-2, Table 49-1). Erosive esophagitis is not seen in eosinophilic esophagitis in its classic form. Recent reports have documented the histologic findings of eosinophilic esophagitis in patients with "normal" esophageal mucosa at endoscopy, which obviously may be found in gastroesophageal reflux disease.

Table 49-1

Endoscopic Findings in Eosinophilic Esophagitis

Feline Esophagus
Concentric multiple rings
Corrugations
Furrows
Granularity
Crepe paper
Normal

Some of the difficulties in differentiating eosinophilic esophagitis from gastroesophageal reflux disease comes from the results of a single-center observational study of 26 patients prospectively followed with a diagnosis of eosinophilic esophagitis. Eighteen men and 8 women aged 17 to 66 were followed. Seventeen out of 26 (66%) had food impactions and 17 carried a diagnosis of GERD. Eleven had previous esophageal dilatations; some with improvement. All had been treated with proton pump inhibitors prior to diagnosis and one had a fundoplication for presumed GERD. The endoscopic findings described above were reported in variable frequency and 6 reported as normal. Pathology demonstrated eosinophilia with higher density in the distal than proximal esophagus, however biopsies had a range of 0.2 to 109 per high power field. pH studies were performed in 24 with 10 (41%) abnormal. Esophageal manometry was completely normal in all but 1 patient (esophageal body motility) whereas 8 had a low lower esophageal sphincter (LES) pressure. As ultimately these patients had failed PPI therapy, the diagnosis of reflux disease was felt to be a cofactor.

Because of the frequency of GERD in the general population, it is entirely unclear whether the presence of an abnormal pH study is indicative of coexistent GERD, suggesting GERD as a cause of eosinophilic esophagitis, a cofactor, or a situation that is completely unrelated. In reality, the clinician is faced with a dilemma common in clinical practice. Eosinophilic esophagitis is an emerging disease with a classic presentation, being extended to unusual and atypical presentations. GERD, a common disease in the adult population, also presents with varying presentations, including dysphagia, and may therefore create problems in differentiation. A careful history, a reliable and thorough endoscopic evaluation with at least 5 esophageal biopsies from both distal and proximal esophagus, and a pathologist familiar with both diseases will help differentiate. Unfortunately, in the clinical practice of gastroenterology, many patients will be treated for both diseases in concert as the long-term outcomes from eosinophilic esophagitis are unclear and many have a recurrent course.

INDEX

Printed in the United States
by Baker & Taylor Publisher Services